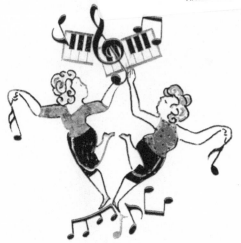

LINE DANCES
75 Dances for 600 Songs

Book Text * Step Sheets
Kitty Russell

Illustrations * Step Sheets
Susan Prats

Copyright 2019
ISBN-978-1-937922-35-1
Published by Kittyco Press
Arlington, Virginia

KITTY

P RESS

NOTE FROM THE AUTHORS

We hope you enjoy this collection of line dances.
Most are easy, for beginners, or people who just want
to dance without having to remember too many steps.

ABOUT THE AUTHORS

Susie Prats and Kitty Russell are retired persons living
in Alexandria and Arlington, Virginia. Both are line
dance enthusiasts. They met in 2015 when Kitty,
recently retired, joined a line dancing class Susie also
attended. Since that time, Susie has become a line
dance instructor and Kitty an occasional choreographer
of line dances.

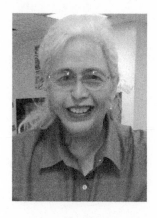
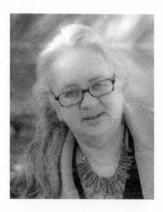

Susan Prats   Kitty Russell

CONTENTS

LINE DANCE BASICS

Walls

Line dancers use the four walls as reference points. Wall 1, or "12 o'clock", or 12:00, is the wall the group faces to start the dance. The wall to the right is "3 o'clock", the wall behind is "6 o'clock", and the wall to the left is "9 o'clock".

Line dances rotate clockwise or counter-clockwise around the walls. "1-wall" dances start and end at 12:00; 2-wall dances start at 12:00 and restart at 6:00; 4-wall dances start at 12:00, then restart at 3:00 or 9:00, then 6:00, then the next wall.

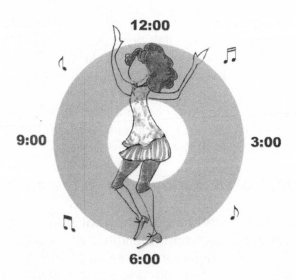

Step direction

Steps can move side-to-side, forward or back, on a diagonal, in a turn, or they can be done in place. When turning, it is helpful to think of the shoulders. A left turn will be in the direction of the left shoulder; a right turn in the direction of the right shoulder.

Dance sequence

Each dance consists of several sets, danced in sequence, over and over until the music stops. Most dances use sets of 8 beats (1-4, 5-8); waltzes use sets of 6 beats (1-3, 4-6).

Variations to the dance sequence

A variation can occur as a step change for a particular set or a restart before finishing a set. There can be an extra set of steps, called a "tag", to keep in time with the music, or to finish facing front (12 o'clock).

Sometimes a dance may be "phrased", with the parts, or "phrases" (A, B, etc.), danced in a particular order (for example, "AABBC, repeat").

Weight, lead and moving with the music

It's important to start at the right point in the music (usually the first beat after the introductory phrase), to move with the music, and to know at all times which foot the weight is on, and which foot will take the next step.

Timing and speed

Different songs have different time signatures. The most common is 4/4 time.

> 4/4 (common) time – 4 quarter notes per measure, with strongest emphasis on 1, then 3.
> --**one**, (two), three, (four)--

> 3/4 (waltz) time - 3 quarter notes per measure, with the emphasis on note 1.
> --**one**, (two), (three)--

> 2/4 time – 2 quarter notes per measure, with the emphasis on note 1.
> --**one**, (two), **one**, (two)--

> 6/8 time – 6 eighth notes per measure, with strongest emphasis on 1, then 4.
> --**one**, (two), (three), four, (five), (six)--

Speed, or tempo, is measured in beats per minute (bpm). 120 bpm is a typical speed for a line dance.

Stepping off the beat

A line dance sequence won't always follow the beat of the music. For example, there may be an extra step between the beats (as with a triple step), or the dancing may be done at half speed, each step taking 2 beats.

Step sheet

The step sheet gives the details of the dance, and the music to dance it to. The step sheet may use abbreviations, "R" for right foot and "L" for left foot and may offer variations of the step pattern as options.

Steps should be danced exactly as described in the step sheet, regardless of how they are usually done.

Steps

Here are short descriptions of steps used for line dancing, some represented in this book and some provided just for reference. Steps can be done in different directions or modified to make a turn.

Dashes are used when steps are off beat (ex: 1-&-2).

Basic:
Step to side, step together, step to side.

Behind-side-cross:
Step behind-step to side-step across.

Brush:
Brush foot forward and upward.

Charleston (4 variations):

Touch forward, step in place, touch back, step in place.

Step forward, touch forward, step back, touch back.

Charleston kick:
Kick forward, step in place, touch back, step in place.

Montana kick:
Step forward, kick forward, step back, touch back.

Coaster:
Step back-together-forward, or
step forward-together-back.

Conga walk:
(forward) Step, step, step forward, point to side.
(back) Step, step, step back, touch.

Elvis knees:
Pop one knee in, then the other, in syncopated pattern
(in, in, in-in-in-in).

Diagonal steps:
Step forward (or back), together, on a diagonal.

Diagonal lock steps:
Step forward (or back), lock behind (or across),
on a diagonal

Flick:
Bend knee and point toes behind.

Heel bounce:
Heels up, heels down.

Hip bump:
Hip to side.

Hitch:
Lift knee up and foot off the floor.

Hook:
Lift foot up and across.

Jazz box:
Step across, step back, step to the side, step together (or across).

K-step:
Step forward diagonal, touch together and clap,
Step back diagonal, touch together and clap,
Step back diagonal, touch together and clap,
Step forward diagonal, touch together and clap.

Kick-ball-change:
Kick-step-step.

Kick-ball-cross:
Kick-step-step across.

Lindy:
Step-together-step to side, rock back, recover.

Mambo:
Rock (in any direction), recover, step together, or rock-recover-step together.

Merengue:
Step to side, together, to side, together.

Monterey 1/4 turn:
Point to side, step together with 1/4 turn (90 degrees), point to other side, step together.

Moon walk:
Slide toe pad back, then heel down.

Night club (or night club two step):
Long step to side, rock back, recover.

Paddle (or pivot):
Step forward, turn and step. Turn can be 1/8 (45 degrees), 1/4 (90 degrees) or 1/2 (180 degrees).

Push step:
Step forward, push together, on a diagonal.

Rhumba:
Step to side, step together, step forward (or back), or step to side-step together-step forward (or back).

Rocking chair:
Rock forward, recover, rock back, recover, or rock back, recover, rock forward, recover.

Sailor:
Step behind-step to side-step to side.

Scissors:
Step to side, step together, step across.

Scuff:
Brush heel against the floor, forward and upward.

Shimmy:
Long step to side, moving shoulders forward and back.

Shuffle box:
Step to side, step together, triple step forward (or back),
step to side, step together, triple step back (or forward).

Skate:
Slide on ball of foot forward diagonal, put heel down
and lift other foot.

Stomp (or stomp up):
Put foot down flat with force (stomp, or, if weight
doesn't change, stomp up).

Sway:
Step to side, while swinging upper body.

Sweep (or ronde):
Slide foot in a circle, front to back or back to front.

Toe fan (one foot)
Toes out, in, out, in.

Toe strut:
Toe touch, heel down.

Triple step:
Step-together-step in any direction or in place.

V-step:
Step forward out, out (shoulder width apart),
step back in, in (together).

Vine:
Step to side, step behind, step to side
(can be done with 1/4 or 1/2 turn;
a rolling vine is with a full turn).

Waltz (or balance):
Long step, step together, step together.

Waltz with turn:
Long step with turn, step together, step together.

Waltz box:
Long step forward (or back), step to side, step together.

Waltz hesitation:
Long step, step together, hold (lifting heels), or
long step, drag together, hold.

Waltz twinkle:
Step across (or behind), step to side, step behind
(or across).

Weave (4 variations):

Step behind, step to side, step across, step to side.

Step across, step to side, step behind, step to side.

Step to side, step behind, step to side, step across.

Step to side, step across, step to side, step behind.

Wizard (or Dorothy or Yellow Brick Road):
Step, lock-step.

Websites

Copperknob is a popular website for step sheets:
https://www.copperknob.co.uk/

Spotify is a website for playing and listening to music:
https://www.spotify.com/us/

Video demonstrations can be found on Copperknob and on YouTube. For example, our reviewer, Debra Ciavarella, offers demonstrations on her channel for Rising Sun Dancers:
https://www.youtube.com/user/ResonantSun17.

THE DANCES

The following pages contain step sheets for the dances, one per page.

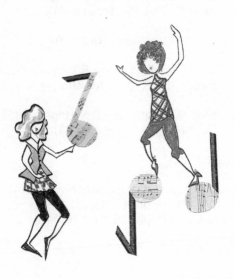

A Kiss to Build a Dream on by Louis Armstrong
KR, 32 count, 4 wall, left lead
Start at vocals "Give me a kiss..."

SHUFFLE BOX LEFT FORWARD, RIGHT BACK

1-2, 3&4	Step L to left (1), step R together (2), triple L (3), R (&), L forward (4)
5-6,7&8	Step R to right (5), step L together (6), triple R (7), L (&), R back (8)

SHUFFLE BOX LEFT FORWARD, RIGHT BACK

1-2, 3&4	Step L to left (1), step R together (2), triple L (3), R (&), L forward (4)
5-6,7&8	Step R to right (5), step L together (6), triple R (7), L (&), R back (8)

SWAY 3, TOUCH, PIVOT 1/8 LEFT X 2

1-4	Sway L (1), R (2), L (3), touch R next to L (4)
5-6	Step R forward (5), pivot 1/8 L (6)
7-8	Step R forward (7), pivot 1/8 L (9:00) (8)

KICK-BALL-CHANGE X 2, SWAY 3, TOUCH

1&2	Kick R forward (1), step on ball of R while raising L (&), step L (2)
3&4	Kick R foot forward (3), step on ball of R while raising L (&), step L (4)
5-8	Sway R (5), L (6), R (7), touch left next to R (8)

Restart

Act Naturally by Buck Owens

KR, 32 count, 2 wall, right lead
Start at vocals "They're gonna put me in the movies..."

CHARLESTON X 2

1-4   Touch R toe forward (1), step R next to L (2),
         touch L toe back (3), step L next to R (4)

5-8   Touch R toe forward (5), step R next to L (6),
         touch L toe back (7), step L next to R (8)

HEEL, HEEL, TRIPLE IN PLACE
HEEL, HEEL, TRIPLE IN PLACE

1-2   Touch R heel to right (1), touch R heel to right (2)
3&4   Triple step, R (3), L (&), R (4) in place

5-6   Touch L heel to left (5), touch L heel to left (6)
7&8   Triple step L (7), R (&), L (8) in place

VINE RIGHT WITH TRIPLE TO RIGHT
VINE LEFT WITH TRIPLE TO LEFT

1-2, 3&4   Step R to right (1), step L behind right (2),
              triple R (3), L (&), R (4) to right
5-6, 7&8   Step L to left (5), step R behind left (6),
              triple L (7), R (&), L (8) to left

WALK 4 WITH 1/2 TURN LEFT
TRIPLE IN PLACE X 2

1-4   Step R (1), L (2), R (3), L (4) forward,
         making 1/2 turn left (6:00)
5&6   Triple step R (5), L (&), R (6) in place
7&8   Triple step L (7), R (&), L (8) in place

Restart

Wall 4: Restart after the Charleston sequences.

Ain't That a Kick in the Head by Dean Martin

KR, 32 count, 2 wall, right lead
Start at vocals "How lucky can one guy be..."

STEP, TOUCH DIAGONAL FORWARD X 4

1-2	Step R to forward right (1), touch L next to R (2)
3-4	Step L to forward left (3), touch R next to L (4)
5-6	Step R to forward right (5), touch L next to R (6)
7-8	Step L to forward left (7), touch R next to L (8)

WALK 3 BACK, KICK
X 2

1-4	Step R (1), L (2), R (3) back, kick L forward (4)
5-8	Step L (5), R (6), L (7) back, kick R forward (8)

VINE RIGHT, TOUCH
VINE LEFT, TOUCH

1-4	Step R to right (1), step L behind R (2), step R to right (3), touch L next to R (4)
5-8	Step L to left (5), step R behind left (6), step L to left (7), touch R next to left (8)

PIVOT 1/8 LEFT X 4

1-2	Step R forward (1), pivot 1/8 L (2)
3-4	Step R forward (3), pivot 1/8 L (4)
5-6	Step R forward (5), pivot 1/8 L (6)
7-8	Step R forward (7), pivot 1/8 L (6:00) (8)

Restart

Ain't Too Proud to Beg, by The Temptations
SP, 32 count, 2 wall, right lead
Start after intro, at vocals, "...ain't too proud to..."

WALK 3 FORWARD, KICK
WALK 3 BACK, TOUCH

1-4   Step R (1), L (2), R (3) forward, kick L (4)
5-8   Step L (5), R (6), L (7) back, touch R next to L (8)

PADDLE 1/4 LEFT X 2

1-2   Step R forward (1), paddle L with 1/4 turn left (9:00) (2)
3-4   Step R forward (3), paddle L with 1/4 turn left (6:00) (4)

VINE RIGHT, TOUCH
VINE LEFT, CROSS
SIDE ROCK, RECOVER, CROSS, HOLD

5-8   Step R to right (5), step L behind R (6),
        step R to right (7), touch L next to R (8)
1-8   Step L to left (1), step R behind L (2), step L to left (3),
        step R across L (4), rock L to left (5), recover R(6),
        step L across R (7), hold (8)

ROCKING CHAIR BACK X 2

1-4   Rock R back (1), step L in place (2),
        rock R forward (3), step L in place (4)
5-8   Rock R back (5), step L in place (6),
        rock R forward (7), step L in place (8)

Restart

All I Do Is Dream of You by Michael Bublé
KR, 32 count, 2 wall, right lead
Start after 16 beats of introductory music, just ahead of vocals

RHUMBA RIGHT BACK, HOLD
RHUMBA LEFT FORWARD, HOLD

1-4   Step R to right (1), step L together (2),
         step R back (3), hold (4)

5-8   Step L to left (5), step R together (6),
         step L forward (7), hold (8)

VINE RIGHT, CROSS
SIDE ROCK, RECOVER, CROSS, HOLD

1-4   Step R to right (1), step L behind R (2),
         step R to right (3), cross L over R (4)
5-8   Rock R to right (5), recover L (6),
         step R across L (7), hold (8)

VINE LEFT, CROSS
SIDE ROCK, RECOVER, CROSS, HOLD

1-4   Step L to left (1), step R behind L (2),
         step L to left (3), cross R over L (4)

5-8   Rock L to left (5), recover R (6),
         cross L over R (7), hold (8)

ROCKING CHAIR
PIVOT 1/4 LEFT X 2

1-4   Rock R forward (1), step L in place (2),
         rock R back (3), step L in place (4)

5-6   Step R forward (5), pivot 1/4 L (9:00) (6)
7-8   Step R forward (7), pivot 1/4 L (6:00) (8)

Restart

All My Exes Live in Texas by George Strait
KR, 32 count, 1 wall, right lead
Start at vocals "All my exes …"

LOCK STEPS FORWARD RIGHT, BRUSH
LOCK STEPS FORWARD LEFT, BRUSH

1-4   Step R diagonally forward to right (1), lock L behind R (2),
        step R diagonally forward to right (3), brush L next to R (4)

5-8   Step L diagonally forward to left (5), lock R behind L (6),
        step L diagonally forward to left (7), brush R next to L (8)

SLOW JAZZ BOX WITH 1/4 TURN RIGHT

1-2   Step R across L (1-2)
3-4   Step L back making 1/4 turn right (3:00) (3-4)
5-6   Step R to right (5-6)
7-8   Step L across R (7-8)

VINE RIGHT, TOUCH
VINE LEFT WITH 1/4 TURN LEFT, TOUCH

1-4   Step R to right (1), step L behind R (2),
        step R to right (3), touch L next to R (4)

5-8   Step L to left (5), step R behind L (6), step L to left
        making 1/4 turn left (12:00) (7), touch R next to L (8)

SCISSORS RIGHT, HOLD
SCISSORS LEFT, HOLD

1-4   Step R to right (1), step L next to R (2),
        cross R over L (3), hold (4)

5-8   Step L to left (5), step R next to L (6),
        cross L over R (7), hold (8)

Restart

Anything Goes by Frank Sinatra
KR, 32 count, 4 wall, right lead
Start at vocals "In olden days…"

BASIC RIGHT, TOUCH
STEP, TOUCH X 2

1-4   Step R to right (1), step L together (2),
        step R to right (3), touch L next to R (4)
5-6   Step L to left (5), touch R next to L (6)
7-8   Step R to right (7), touch L next to R (8)

BASIC LEFT, TOUCH
STEP, TOUCH X 2

1-4   Step L to left (1), step R together (2),
        step L to left (3), touch R next to L (4)
5-6   Step R (5), touch L next to R (6)
7-8   Step L (7), touch R next to L (8)

RHUMBA RIGHT BACK, HOLD
RHUMBA LEFT FORWARD, HOLD

1-4   Step R to right (1), step L together (2),
        step R back (3), hold (4)

5-8   Step L to left (5), step R together (6),
        step L forward (7), hold (8)

ROCKING CHAIR
PIVOT 1/8 LEFT X 2

1-4   Rock R forward (1), step L in place (2),
        rock R back (3), step L in place (4)

5-6   Step R forward (5), pivot 1/8 L (6)
7-8   Step R forward (7), pivot 1/8 L (9:00) (8)

Restart

(Baby) Hully Gully by The Olympics
SP, 16 count, 4 wall, right lead
Start 8 beats in

LINDY RIGHT
LINDY LEFT WITH 1/4 TURN RIGHT

1&2, 3-4   Triple step R (1), L (&), R (2) to right,
        rock L behind R (3), recover R (4)

5&6, 7-8   Triple step L (5), R (&), L to left (6),
        rock R behind L making 1/4 turn right (3:00) (7),
        recover L (8)

JAZZ BOX
STEP, TOUCH X 2

1-4 Step R across L (1), step L back (2),
   step R to right (3), step L next to R (4)

5-6 Step R (5), touch L (6)
7-8 Step L (7), touch R (8)

Restart

Be My Baby by The Ronettes
KR, 16 count, 4 wall, right lead
Start 16 beats in

BASIC RIGHT, TOUCH
STEP, TOUCH X 2

1-4   Step R to right (1), step L together (2),
         step R to right (3), touch L next to R (4)
5-6   Step L to left (5), touch R next to L (6)
7-8   Step R to right (7), touch L next to R (8)

LINDY LEFT

1&2, 3-4   Triple step L (1), R (&), L (2) to left,
         rock R back (3), recover L (4)

PIVOT 1/8 LEFT X 2

5-6   Step R forward (5), pivot 1/8 L (6)
7-8   Step R forward (7), pivot 1/8 L (9:00) (8)

Restart

Begin the Beguine by Richard Clayderman
SP, 16 count, 4 wall, right lead
Start 24 beats into music

RHUMBA RIGHT FORWARD, TOUCH
RHUMBA LEFT BACK WITH DRAG

1-4   Step R to right (1), step L together (2),
         step R forward (3), touch L next to R (4)

5-8   Step L to left (5), step R together (6),
         step L back (7), drag R together (8)

RIGHT BACK, RECOVER, TRIPLE FORWARD
LEFT FORWARD, 1/4 TURN RIGHT, CROSS TRIPLE TO RIGHT

1-2, 3&4   Rock R back (1), recover L (2),
               triple R (3), L (&), R (4) forward

5-6, 7&8   Step L forward (5),
               step R with 1/4 turn right (3:00)(6),
               cross triple L (7), R (&), L (8) to right

Restart

Blue Bayou by Linda Ronstadt

SP, 32 count, 4 wall, right lead
Begin 16 beats into music

SHUFFLE BOX RIGHT FORWARD, LEFT BACK
X 2

1-2, 3&4	Step R to right (1), L together (2), triple R (3), L (&), R (4) forward
5-6, 7&8	Step L to left (5), R together (6), triple L (7), R (&), L (8) back
1-2, 3&4	Step R to right (1), L together (2), triple R (3), L (&), R (4) forward
5-6, 7&8	Step L to left (5), R together (6), triple L (7), R (&), L (8) back

ROCK BACK, RECOVER, TRIPLE FORWARD
ROCK FORWARD, RECOVER, TRIPLE BACK

1-2, 3&4	Rock R back (1), recover L (2), triple R (3), L (&), R (4) forward
5-6, 7&8	Rock L forward (5), recover R (6), triple L (7), R (&), L (8) back

JAZZ BOX WITH 1/8 TURN RIGHT
JAZZ BOX WITH 1/8 TURN RIGHT

1-4	Step R across L (1), step L back (2), step R to right making 1/8 turn right (3), step L next to R (4)
5-8	Step R across L (5), step L back (6), step R to right making 1/8 turn right (3:00) (7), step L next to R (8)

Restart

Blueberry Hill by Fats Domino
KR, 32 count, 4 wall, right lead
Start 16 beats in, at vocals, "I've found my freedom..."

SHUFFLE BOX RIGHT BACK, LEFT FORWARD
1-2, 3&4   Step R to right (1), step L together (2),
                       triple step R (3), L (&), R (4) back

5-6, 7&8   Step L to left (5), step R together (6),
                       triple step L (7), R (&), L (8) forward

TRIPLE WITH 1/8 TURN LEFT X 2
JAZZ BOX WITH 1/4 TURN RIGHT
1&2   Triple step R (1), L (&), R (2) with 1/8 turn left
3&4   Triple step L (3), R (&), L (4) with 1/8 turn left (9:00)

5-8   Step R across L (5), step L back (6),
            step R to right turning 1/4 right (12:00) (7),
            step L next to R (8)

TRIPLE WITH 1/8 TURN LEFT X 4
1&2   Triple step R (1), L (&), R (2) with 1/8 turn left
3&4   Triple step L (3), R (&), L (4) with 1/8 turn left
5&6   Triple step R (5), L (&), R (6) with 1/8 turn left
7&8   Triple step L (7), R (&), L (8) with 1/8 turn left (6:00)

JAZZ BOX WITH 1/4 TURN RIGHT
STEP, TOUCH X 2
1-4   Step R across L (1), step L back (2), step R to right
            turning 1/4 right (9:00) (3), step L next to R (4)

5-6   Step R to right (5), touch L next to R (6)
7-8   Step L to left (7), touch R next to L (8)

Restart

Option: Replace triples with pivots 1/8 L.

Boy from NYC by The Ad Libs

SP, 16 count, 2 wall, right lead
Start 32 beats into music

**MAMBO FORWARD, MAMBO BACK
MAMBO RIGHT, MAMBO LEFT**

1&2	Rock R forward (1), recover L (&), step R next to L (2)
3&4	Rock L back (3), recover R (&), step L next to R (4)
5&6	Rock R to right (5), recover L (&), step R next to L (6)
7&8	Rock L to left (7), recover R (&), step L next to R (8)

PADDLE 1/8 LEFT X 4

1&	Step R forward (1), paddle 1/8 L (&)
2&	Step R forward (2), paddle 1/8 L (&)
3&	Step R forward (3), paddle 1/8 L (&)
4&	Step R forward (4), paddle 1/8 L (6:00) (&)

ROCKING CHAIR X 2

5&6&	Rock R forward (5), step L in place (&), rock R back (6), step L in place (&)
7&8&	Rock R forward (7), step L in place (&), rock R back (8), step L in place (&)

Restart

Option: Replace 2 fast rocking chairs with
1 rocking chair at regular speed (5-8).

Breaking Up Is Hard To Do by Neil Sedaka
SP, 32 count, 4 wall, right lead
Start after 32 beats at vocals "...love away from me..."

SHUFFLE BOX RIGHT FORWARD, LEFT BACK

1-2,3&4	Step R to right (1), step L together (2), triple R (3), L (&), R (4) forward
5-6,7&8	Step L to left (5), step R together (7), triple L (7), R (&), L (8) back

STEP, BRUSH, STEP, BRUSH, VINE RIGHT, TOUCH

1-2	Step R (1), brush L (2)
3-4	Step L (3), brush R (4)
5-8	Step R to right (5), step L behind R (6), step R to right (7), touch L next to R (8)

VINE LEFT WITH 1/4 TURN LEFT, TOUCH
STEP, BRUSH, STEP, BRUSH

1-4	Step L to left (1), step R behind L (2), step L to left making 1/4 turn left (9:00) (3), touch R next to L (4)
5-6	Step R (5), brush L (6)
7-8	Step L (7), brush R (8)

V-STEP, HIP BUMP RIGHT, RIGHT, LEFT, LEFT

1-2	Step R to forward right (1), step L to forward left (2)
3-4	Step R back to center (3), step L next to R (4)
5-6	Hip bump right (5), hip bump right (6)
7-8	Hip bump left (7), hip bump left (8)

Restart

Tag: After wall 3, add hip bumps, R, R, L, L.

Button Up Your Overcoat
by Miss Rose and her Rhythm Percolators
KR, 16 count, 2 wall, right lead
Start at vocals "Listen, big boy…"

CHARLESTON X 2

1-4	Touch R toe forward (1), step R next to L (2), touch L toe back (3), step L next to R (4)
5-8	Touch R toe forward (5), step R next to L (6), touch L toe back (7), step L next to R (8)

SAILOR X 2

1&2	Step R behind L (1), step L to left (&), step R to right (2)
3&4	Step L behind R (3), step R to right (&), step L to left (4)

PIVOT 1/4 LEFT X 2

5-6	Step R forward (5), pivot 1/4 L (9:00) (6)
7-8	Step R forward (7), pivot 1/4 L (6:00) (8)

Restart

C'est Magnifique by Dean Martin
KR, 32 count, 4 wall, right lead
Start at vocals "When love comes in…"

RHUMBA RIGHT FORWARD, TOUCH
RHUMBA LEFT BACK, TOUCH

1-4   Step R to right (1), step L together (2),
        step R forward (3), touch L next to R (4)
5-8   Step L to left (5), step R together (6),
        step L back (7), touch R next to L (8)

VINE RIGHT, TOUCH
VINE LEFT, CROSS
SIDE ROCK, RECOVER, CROSS, HOLD

1-4   Step R to right (1), step L behind right (2),
        step R to right (3), touch L next to R (4)
5-8   Step L to left (5), step R behind L (6),
        step L to left (7), cross R over L (8)
1-4   Rock L to left (1), recover R (2),
        cross L over R (3), hold (4)

ROCKING CHAIR X 2

5-8   Rock R forward (5), step L in place (6),
        rock R back (7), step L in place (8)
1-4   Rock R forward (1), step L in place (2),
        rock R back (3), step L in place (4)

JAZZ BOX WITH 1/4 TURN RIGHT

5-8   Step R across L (5), step L back (6),
        step R to right turning 1/4 right (3:00) (7),
        step L next to R (8)

Restart

Cab Driver by The Mills Brothers
KR, 32 count, 4 wall, right lead
Start after 8 beats of intro music

LOCK STEPS FORWARD RIGHT, BRUSH
LOCK STEPS FORWARD LEFT, HITCH

1-4   Step R diagonally forward to right (1), lock L behind R (2), step R diagonally forward to right (3), brush L (4)

5-8   Step L diagonally forward to left (5), lock R behind L (6), step L diagonally forward to left (7), hitch R knee up with a little kick (8)

STEP BACK, HITCH
X 4

1-2   Step R back (1), hitch L knee up with a little kick (2)
3-4   Step L back (3), hitch R knee up with a little kick (4)
5-6   Step R back (5), hitch L knee up with a little kick (6)
7-8   Step L back (7), hitch R knee up with a little kick (8)

VINE RIGHT, TOUCH
VINE LEFT WITH 1/4 TURN LEFT, TOUCH

1-4   Step R to right (1), step L behind R (2), step R to right (3), touch L next to R (4)
5-8   Step L to left (5), step R behind L (6), step L to left making 1/4 turn left (9:00) (7), touch R next to L (8)

SCISSORS RIGHT, HOLD
SCISSORS LEFT, HOLD

1-4   Step R to right (1), step L next to R (2), cross R over L (3), hold (4)
5-8   Step L to left (5), step R next to L (6), cross L over R (7), hold (8)

Restart

Chapel of Love by The Dixie Cups

SP, 32 count, 4 wall, right lead
Start at vocals, 56 beats into music

WALK 3 FORWARD, POINT LEFT
WALK 3 BACK, HITCH

1-4 Walk forward R (1), L (2), R (3), point L to side (4)
5-8 Walk back L (5), R (6), L (7), hitch R (8)

POINT RIGHT OUT, IN, OUT, IN
VINE RIGHT, TOUCH

1-4 Point R out to right (1), in (2), out (3), in (4)
5-8 Step R to right (5), step L behind R (6),
step R to right (7), touch L next to R (8)

POINT LEFT OUT, IN, OUT, IN
VINE LEFT WITH 1/4 TURN LEFT, TOUCH

1-4 Point L out to left (1), in (2), out (3), in (4)
5-8 Step L to left (5), step R behind L (6),
step L to left making 1/4 turn L (9:00) (7),
touch R next to L (8)

K-STEP WITH CLAPS

1-2 Step R to right forward diagonal (1),
touch L next to R and clap (2)
3-4 Step L to left back diagonal (3),
touch R next to L and clap (4)
5-6 Step R to right back diagonal (5),
touch left next to R and clap (6)
7-8 Step L to left forward diagonal (7),
touch R next to L and clap (8)

Restart

Chihuahua by DJ BoBo
KR, 16 count, 4 wall, right lead
Start 16 beats in, when music ratchets up a notch

MAMBO RIGHT, MAMBO LEFT

1&2   Rock R to right (1), recover L (&),
        step R next to L (2)

3&4   Rock L to left (3), recover R (&),
        step L next to R (4)

ROCK FORWARD, RECOVER, TRIPLE BACK
ROCK BACK, RECOVER, TRIPLE FORWARD

5-6, 7&8   Rock R forward (5), recover L (6),
                triple step R (7), L (&), R (8) back
1-2, 3&4   Rock L back (1), recover R (2),
                triple step L (3), R (&), L (4) forward

JAZZ BOX WITH 1/4 TURN RIGHT

5-8   Step R across L (5), step L back (6),
        step R to right turning 1/4 right (3:00) (7),
        step L next to R (8)

Restart

Dance, Dance, Dance by The Beach Boys

SP, 56 count, 4 wall, right lead
Start at vocals "…After six hours of school…"

JAZZ BOX WITH 1/8 TURN RIGHT X 2
1-4   Step R across L (1), step L back (2), step R to right
        turning 1/8 right (3), step L next to R (4)
5-8   Step R across L (5), step L back (6), step R to right
        turning 1/8 right (3:00) (7), step L next to R (8)
V-STEP X 2
1-2   Step R to forward right (1), step L to forward left (2)
3-4   Step R back to center (3), step L next to R (4)
5-6   Step R to forward right (5), step L to forward left (6)
7-8   Step R back to center (7), step L next to R (8)
BASIC RIGHT, FLICK, BASIC LEFT, FLICK
1-4   Step R to right (1), step L together (2), step R to right (3),
        flick L (4)
5-8   Step L to left (5), step R together (6), step L to left (7),
        flick R (8)
BASIC RIGHT, FLICK, BASIC LEFT, FLICK
1-4   Step R to right (1), step L together (2), step R to right (3),
        flick L (4)
5-8   Step L to left (5), step R together (6), step L to left (7),
        flick R (8)
DIAGONAL STEPS FORWARD RIGHT, HITCH
DIAGONAL STEPS FORWARD LEFT, HITCH
1-4   Step R (1), L (2), R (3) diagonally forward to right,
        hitch L (4)
5-8   Step L (5), R (6), L (7) diagonally forward to left,
        hitch R (8)
DIAGONAL STEPS BACK RIGHT, HITCH
DIAGONAL STEPS BACK LEFT, HITCH
1-4   Step R (1), L (2), R (3) diagonally back to right,
        hitch L (4)
5-8   Step L (5), R (6), L (7) diagonally back to left,
        hitch R (8)
BASIC RIGHT, FLICK, BASIC LEFT, BRUSH
1-4   Step R to right (1), step L together (2), step R to right (3),
        flick L (4)
5-8   Step L to left (5), step R together (6), step L to left (7),
        brush R (8)
Restart

Dancing in the Street by Martha Reeves & The Vandellas
SP, 48 count, 2 wall, right lead
Start 48 beats in

MONTEREY 1/4 TURN RIGHT, JAZZ BOX
1-2   Point R to right (1), step R next to L
        making 1/4 turn right (3:00) (2)
3-4   Point L to left (3), step L next to R (4)
5-8   Step R across L (5), step L back (6),
        step R to right (7), step L next to R (8)

MONTEREY 1/4 TURN RIGHT, JAZZ BOX
1-2   Point R to right (1), step R next to L
        making 1/4 turn right (6:00) (2)
3-4   Point L to left (3), step L next to R (4)
5-8   Step R across L (5), step L back (6),
        step R to right (7), step L next to R (8)

WALK 3 FORWARD, KICK AND CLAP
WALK 3 BACK, TOUCH
1-4   Step R (1), L (2), R (3) forward, kick L and clap (4)
5-8   Step L (5), R (6), L (7) back, touch R next to L (8)

LINDY RIGHT, LINDY LEFT
1&2, 3-4   Triple step R (1), L (&), R (2) to right,
        rock L back (3), recover R (4)
5&6, 7-8   Triple step L (5), R (&), L (6) to left,
        rock R back (7), recover L (8)

Restart

Option: In section 3, "dust off" at count 8 by slapping palms across thighs, R palm across R thigh and L palm across L thigh.

Danke Schoen by Wayne Newton
KR, 16 count, 4 wall, right lead
Start 8 beats in, with vocals

RHUMBA RIGHT FORWARD
RHUMBA LEFT FORWARD

1&2   Step R to right (1), step L together (&),
        step R forward (2)
3&4   Step L to left (3), step R together (&),
        step L forward (4)

RHUMBA RIGHT BACK
RHUMBA LEFT BACK

5&6   Step R to right (5), step L together (&),
        step R back (6)
7&8   Step L to left (7), step R together (&),
        step L back (8)

MAMBO RIGHT
MAMBO LEFT

1&2   Rock R to right (1) recover L (&),
        step R next to L (2)
3&4   Rock L to left (3), recover R (&),
        step L next to R (4)

SLOW JAZZ BOX WITH 1/4 TURN RIGHT

5-8   Step R across L (5),
        step L back making 1/4 turn right (3:00) (6),
        step R to right (7), step L next to R (8)

Restart

Do Ya' by K. T. Oslin
KR, 16 count, 4 wall, left lead
Start at vocals "Do you still get a thrill…"

RHUMBA LEFT FORWARD
RHUMBA RIGHT BACK

1&2   Step L to left (1), step R next to L (&),
        step L forward (2)

3&4   Step R to right (3), step L next to R (&),
        step R back (4)

WALK 2 BACK, COASTER

5-6   Step L back (5), step R back (6)
7&8   Step L back (7), step R next to L (&),
        step L forward (8)

SCISSORS RIGHT, SCISSORS LEFT

1&2   Step R to right (1), step L next to R (&),
        cross R over L (2)

3&4   Step L to left (3), step R next to L (&),
        cross L over R (4)

PIVOT 1/4 LEFT
TRIPLE IN PLACE

5-6   Step R forward (5), pivot 1/4 L (9:00) (6)
7&8   Triple step R (7), L (&), R (8) in place

Restart

Don't Get Around Much Anymore by Anne Murray

KR, 32 count, 4 wall, right lead
Start at vocals "When I'm not playing solitaire…"

SLOW CHARLESTON (each step to 2 beats of music)
1-2   Touch R toe forward (1-2)
3-4   Step R next to L (3-4)
5-6   Touch L toe back (5-6)
7-8   Step L next to R (7-8)

SLOW CHARLESTON (each step to 2 beats of music)
1-2   Touch R toe forward (1-2)
3-4   Step R next to L (3-4)
5-6   Touch L toe back (5-6)
7-8   Step L next to R (7-8)

BASIC RIGHT, TOUCH, BASIC LEFT, TOUCH
1-4   Step R to right (1), step L together (2), step R to right (3), touch L next to R (4)

5-8   Step L to left (5), step R together (6), step L to left (7), touch R next to L (8)

ROCKING CHAIR WITH 1/8 TURN LEFT X 2
1-4   Rock R forward (1), step L in place (2), rock R back making 1/8 turn left (3), step L in place (4)

5-8   Rock R forward (5), step L in place (6), rock R back making 1/8 turn left (9:00) (7), step L in place (8)

Restart

Option: Replace 2 rocking chairs with 1 slow rocking chair:
1-8   Rock R forward (1-2), step L in place (3-4), rock R back making 1/4 turn left (9:00) (5-6), step L in place (7-8)

Don't It Make My Brown Eyes Blue by Crystal Gayle

SP, 32 count, 4 wall, right lead
Begin 16 beats into music

VINE RIGHT, TOUCH ACROSS
STEP, TOUCH ACROSS, STEP, TOUCH ACROSS

1-4	Step R to right (1), step L behind R (2), step R to right (3), touch L over R (4)
5-6	Step L (5), touch R over L (6)
7-8	Step R (7), touch L over R (8)

VINE LEFT, TOUCH ACROSS
STEP, TOUCH ACROSS, STEP, TOUCH ACROSS

1-4	Step L to left (1), step R behind left (2), step L to left (3), cross touch R over L (4)
5-6	Step R (5), touch L over R (6)
7-8	Step L (7), touch R over L (8)

PADDLE 1/4 LEFT X 2
JAZZ BOX WITH 1/4 TURN RIGHT

1-2	Step R forward (1), paddle 1/4 L (9:00) (2)
3-4	Step R forward (3), paddle 1/4 L (6:00) (4)
5-8	Step R across L (5), step L back (6), step R to right turning 1/4 right (9:00) (7), step L next to R (8)

TRIPLE FORWARD X 2, SWAY (4)

1&2	Triple R (1), L (&), R (2) forward
3&4	Triple L (3), R (&), L (4) forward
5-8	Sway R (5), L (6), R (7), L (8)

Restart

Duke of Earl by Gene Chandler
KR, 32 count, 4 wall, right lead
Start with vocals, "…I walk through this world…"

MERENGUE RIGHT 7, TOUCH
LINDY LEFT
ROCKING CHAIR

1-2	Step R to right (1), step L next to R (2)
3-4	Step R to right (3), step L next to R (4)
5-6	Step R to right (5), step L next to R (6)
7-8	Step R to right (7), touch L next to R (8)

1&2, 3-4	Triple step L (1), R (&), L (2) to left, rock R back (3), recover L (4)

5-8	Rock R forward (5), step L in place (6), rock R back (7), step L in place (8)

TRIPLE WITH 1/8 TURN LEFT X 2

1&2	Triple step R (1), L (&), R (2) with 1/8 turn left
3&4	Triple step L (3), R (&), L (4) with 1/8 turn left (9:00)

LINDY RIGHT, LINDY LEFT

5&6, 7-8	Triple step R (5), L (&), R (6) to right, rock L back (7), recover R (8)
1&2, 3-4	Triple step L (1), R (&), L (2) to left, rock R back (3), recover L (4)

KICK-BALL-CHANGE X 2

5&6	Kick R forward (5), step on ball of R while raising L (&), step L (6)
7&8	Kick R foot forward (7), step on ball of R while raising L (&), step L (8)

Restart

Everybody's Somebody's Fool by Connie Francis
KR,16 count, 4 wall, right lead
Start 32 beats in, at vocals

RHUMBA RIGHT FORWARD
RHUMBA LEFT BACK

1&2	Step R to right (1), step L together (&), step R forward (2)
3&4	Step L to left (3), step R together (&), step L back (4)

MAMBO RIGHT, MAMBO LEFT

5&6	Rock R to right (5), recover L (&), step R next to L (6)
7&8	Rock L to left (7), recover R (&), step L next to R (8)

PIVOT 1/8 LEFT X 4

1&	Step R forward (1), pivot 1/8 L (&)
2&	Step R forward (2), pivot 1/8 L (&)
3&	Step R forward (3), pivot 1/8 L (&)
4&	Step R forward (4), pivot 1/8 L (6:00) (&)

SLOW JAZZ BOX WITH 1/4 TURN RIGHT

5-8	Step R across L (5), step L back making 1/4 turn right (9:00) (6), step R to right (7), step L next to R (8)

Restart

Option: Replace 4 pivots with 2 slow pivots:
1-2 Step R forward (1), pivot 1/4 L (9:00) (2)
3-4 Step R forward (3), pivot 1/4 L (6:00) (4)

Family Tradition by Hank Williams, Jr.
KR, 32 count, 2 wall, right lead
Start at vocals "Country music singers..."

LOCK STEPS FORWARD RIGHT, BRUSH
LOCK STEPS FORWARD LEFT, TOUCH

1-4	Step R diagonally forward to right (1), lock L behind R (2), step R diagonally forward right (3), brush L next to R (4)
5-8	Step L diagonally forward to left (5), lock R behind L (6), step L diagonally forward to left (7), touch R next to L (8)

WALK 3 BACK, HITCH
X 2

1-4	Step R (1), L(2), R (3) back hitch L knee up with a little kick (4)
5-8	Step L (5), R 6), L (7) back, hitch R knee up with a little kick (8)

VINE RIGHT, TOUCH, VINE LEFT, TOUCH

1-4	Step R to right (1), step L behind right (2), step R to right (3), touch L next to R (4)
5-8	Step L to left (5), step R behind L (6), step L to left (7), touch R next to L (8)

STEP, TOUCH X 4 WITH 1/2 TURN LEFT

1-2	Step R (1), touch L (2) making 1/8 turn left
3-4	Step L (3), touch R (4) making 1/8 turn left
5-6	Step R (5), touch L (6) making 1/8 turn left
7-8	Step L (7), touch R (8) making 1/8 turn left (6:00)

Restart

Tag: After even walls (2, 4, etc.), add 2 step, touches.

Option: Replace vine/touches with lindys.

Fascination by Al Martino
SP, 24 count, 4 wall, left lead, *waltz*
Start at vocals, after intro music

LEFT TWINKLE, RIGHT TWINKLE WITH 1/4 TURN RIGHT

1-3   Step L across R (1), step R to right (2),
        step L slightly back behind R (3)
4-6   Step R across L (4), step L to left (5),
        step R slightly back making 1/4 turn right (3:00) (6)

LEFT TWINKLE, RIGHT TWINKLE

1-3   Step L across R (1), step R to right (2),
        step L slightly back behind R (3)
4-6   Step R across L (4), step L to left (5),
        step R slightly back behind L (6)

WALTZ FORWARD TO RIGHT DIAGONAL
WALTZ BACK

1-3   Long step L forward to right diagonal (1),
        step R together (2), step L in place (3)
4-6   Long step R back to center (4), step L together (5),
        step R in place (6)

WALTZ FORWARD TO LEFT DIAGONAL
WALTZ BACK

1-3   Long step L forward to left diagonal (1), step R together
(2),
        step L in place (3)
4-6   Long step R back to center (4), step L together (5),
        step R in place (6)

Restart

Forever and Ever Amen by Randy Travis
KR, 32 count, 4 wall, right lead
Start 8 beats in at vocals, "You may think that…"

SHUFFLE BOX RIGHT FORWARD, LEFT BACK
1-2,3&4   Step R to right (1), step L together (2),
                  triple R (3), L (&), R (4) forward

5-6,7&8   Step L to left (5), step R together (7),
                  triple L (7), R (&), L (8) back

LINDY RIGHT
LINDY LEFT WITH 1/4 TURN RIGHT
1&2, 3-4   Triple step R (1), L (&), R (2) to right,
                  rock L behind R (3), recover R (4)
5&6, 7-8   Triple step L (5), R (&), L to left (6),
                  rock R behind L making 1/4 turn right (3:00) (7),
                  recover L (8)

JAZZ BOX WITH 1/4 TURN RIGHT
ROCKING CHAIR
1-4   Step R across L (1), step L back (2),
           step R to right turning 1/4 right (6:00) (3),
           step L next to R (4)

5-8   Rock R forward (5), step L in place (6),
           rock R back (7), step L in place (8)

TRIPLE FORWARD X 2
JAZZ BOX WITH 1/4 TURN RIGHT
1&2   Triple step R (1), L (&), R (2) forward
3&4   Triple step L (3), R (&), L (4) forward

5-8   Step R across L (5), step L back (6),
           step R to right turning 1/4 right (9:00) (7),
           step L next to R (8)

Restart

Wall 5: Restart halfway through, just before first jazz box.
Option: Replace shuffle box with a rhumba box.

Gentle on My Mind by The Band Perry
KR, 32 count, 2 wall, right lead
Start 8 beats in at vocals

SHUFFLE BOX RIGHT FORWARD, LEFT BACK
1-2, 3&4   Step R to right (1), L together (2),
            triple R (3), L (&), R (4) forward
5-6, 7&8   Step L to left (5), R together (6),
            triple L (7), R (&), L (8) back

BACK, BACK, TRIPLE BACK
BACK, FORWARD, TRIPLE FORWARD
1-2   Step R back (1), L back (2)
3&4   Triple R (3), L (&), R (4) back
5-6   Step L back (5), R forward (6)
7&8   Triple L (7), R (&), L (8) forward

ROCK RIGHT, RECOVER, CROSS TRIPLE TO LEFT
ROCK LEFT, RECOVER, CROSS TRIPLE TO RIGHT
1-2, 3&4   Rock R to right (1), recover L (2),
            triple R across L (3), L (&), R across L (4)
5-6, 7&8   Rock L to left (5), recover R (6),
            triple L across R (7), R (&), L across R (8)

PIVOT 1/8 LEFT X 4
1-2   Step R forward (1), pivot 1/8 L (2)
3-4   Step R forward (3), pivot 1/8 L (4)
5-6   Step R forward (5), pivot 1/8 L (6)
7-8   Step R forward (7), pivot 1/8 L (6:00) (8)

Restart

Tag: After even walls add a shuffle box, forward and back.

Option: Replace pivots with triples:
1&2   Triple step R (1), L (&), R (2) with 1/8 turn left
3&4   Triple step L (3), R (&), L (4) with 1/8 turn left
5&6   Triple step R (5), L (&), R (6) with 1/8 turn left
7&8   Triple step L (7), R (&), L (8) with 1/8 turn left (6:00)

Glow Worm by The Mills Brothers
KR, 32 count, 2 wall, left lead
Start at vocals "Shine little glow worm, glimmer, glimmer…"

RHUMBA LEFT FORWARD, HOLD
RHUMBA RIGHT FORWARD, HOLD
1-4   Step L to left (1), step R together (2),
        step L forward (3), hold (4)

5-8   Step R to right (5), step L together (6),
        step R forward (7), hold (8)

RHUMBA LEFT BACK, HOLD
RHUMBA RIGHT BACK, HOLD
1-4   Step L to left (1), step R together (2),
        step L back (3), hold (4)

5-8   Step R to right (5), step L together (6),
        step R back (7), hold (8)

COASTER, HOLD
PIVOT 1/8 LEFT X 4
MAMBO RIGHT, HOLD
1-4   Step L back (1), step R next to L (2),
        step L forward (3), hold (4)

5-6   Step R forward (5), pivot 1/8 L (6)
7-8   Step R forward (7), pivot 1/8 L (8)
1-2   Step R forward (1), pivot 1/8 L (2)
3-4   Step R forward (3), pivot 1/8 L (6:00) (4)

5-8   Rock R to right (5), recover L (6),
        step R next to L (7), hold (8)

Restart

Option: Replace 4 pivots with 2 slow pivots:
5-8 Step R forward (5-6), pivot 1/4 L (9:00) (7-8)
1-4 Step R forward (1-2), pivot 1/4 L (6:00) (3-4)

Goody, Goody by Ella Fitzgerald

KR, 32 count, 4 wall, right lead
Start at vocals "So, you met someone…"

PUSH STEP 7 FORWARD RIGHT, TOUCH

1-8 Step R (1), push L (2), step R(3), push L(4), step R(5), push L(6), step R (7) all forward right, touch L (8)

STEP, TOUCH DIAGONAL BACK X 4

1-2 Step L to back left (1), touch R next to L (2)
3-4 Step R to back right (3), touch L next to R (4)
5-6 Step L to back left (5), touch R next to L (6)
7-8 Step R to back right (7), touch L next to R (8)

VINE LEFT WITH 1/4 TURN LEFT, TOUCH

1-4 Step L to left (1), step R behind L (2), step L to left making 1/4 turn left (9:00) (3), touch R next to L (4)

STEP RIGHT FORWARD DIAGONAL, TOUCH
STEP LEFT BACK DIAGONAL, TOUCH
ROCK BACK, RECOVER X 4

5-6 Step R diagonally forward right (5), touch L next to R (6)
7-8 Step L diagonally back left (7), touch R next to L (8)

1-2 Rock R diagonally back right (1), recover L (2)
3-4 Rock R diagonally back right (3), recover L (4)
5-6 Rock R diagonally back right (5), recover L (6)
7-8 Rock R diagonally back right (7), recover L (8)

Restart

Harper Valley PTA by Jeannie C. Riley
SP, 32 count, 4 wall, right lead
Start 16 beats into music

WALK 3 FORWARD, TOUCH LEFT
WALK 2 BACK, 1/4 TURN LEFT, HITCH

1-4   Walk R (1), L (2), R (3) forward, touch L to left (4)
5-8   Walk L back (5), R back (6), 1/4 turn L (9:00) (7),
        hitch R knee up (8)

MERENGUE RIGHT 7, TOUCH

1-2   Step R to right (1), slide L next to R (2)
3-4   Step R to right (3), slide L next to R (4)
5-6   Step R to right (5), slide L next to R (6)
7-8   Step R to right (7), touch L next to R (8)

RHUMBA LEFT FORWARD, TOUCH
RHUMBA RIGHT BACK, TOUCH

1-4   Step L to left (1), step R together (2),
        step L forward (3), touch R next to L (4)

5-8   Step R to right (5), step L together (6),
        step R back (7), touch L next to R (8)

VINE LEFT, CROSS
SIDE ROCK, RECOVER, CROSS, HOLD

1-4   Step L to left (1), step R behind L (2),
        step L to left (3), cross R over L (4)

5-8   Rock L to left (5), recover R (6),
        cross L over R (7), hold (8)

Restart

Heaven's Just a Sin Away by The Kendalls
KR, 16 count, 2 wall, right lead
Start at vocals "Heaven's just a sin away..."

LOCK STEPS FORWARD RIGHT
LOCK STEPS FORWARD LEFT

1&2 Step R diagonally forward to right (1), lock L behind R (&),
   step R diagonally forward to right (2)

3&4 Step L diagonally forward to left (3), lock R behind L (&),
   step L diagonally forward to left (4)

WALK 4 BACK

5-8 Step R (5), L (6), R (7), L (8) back

SCISSORS RIGHT, SCISSORS LEFT

1&2 Step R to right (1), step L next to R (&),
   cross R over L (2)

3&4 Step L to left (3), step R next to L (&),
   cross L over R (4)

WALK 4 FORWARD WITH 1/2 TURN LEFT

5-8 Step R (5), L (6), R (7), L (8) forward,
   making 1/2 turn left (6:00)

Restart

Tag: After walls 2 and 9, step R, step L.

I Believe in You by Don Williams
KR, 32 count, 2 wall, right lead
Start 32 beats in with vocals

STEP, TOGETHER, TRIPLE FORWARD RIGHT
ROCK FORWARD LEFT, RECOVER,
TRIPLE WITH 1/4 TURN LEFT

1-2, 3&4	Step R diagonally forward right (1), L together (2), triple R (3), L (&), R (4) forward right
5-6, 7&8	Rock L diagonally forward left (5), recover R (6), triple L (7), R (&), L (8) with 1/4 turn left (9:00)

VINE RIGHT WITH TRIPLE TO RIGHT
VINE LEFT WITH 1/4 TURN LEFT AND TRIPLE TO LEFT

1-2, 3&4	Step R to right (1), step L behind right (2), triple R (3), L (&), R (4) to right
5-6, 7&8	Step L to left (5), step R behind left (6), turn 1/4 left (6:00) and triple L (7), R (&), L (8) to left

STEP RIGHT FORWARD DIAGONAL, TOUCH, TRIPLE HOME
ROCK BACK, RECOVER X 2

1-2	Step R diagonally forward right (1), touch L next to R (2)
3&4	Triple step L (3), R (&), L (4) diagonally left back to home
5-6	Rock R diagonally back right (5), recover L (6)
7-8	Rock R diagonally back right (7), recover L (8)

TRIPLE WITH 1/8 TURN LEFT X 2
JAZZ BOX WITH 1/4 TURN RIGHT

1&2	Triple R (1), L (&), R (2) forward making 1/8 turn left
3&4	Triple L (3), R (&), L (4) to left making 1/8 turn left (3:00)
5-8	Step R across L (5), step L back (6), step R to right turning 1/4 right (6:00) (7), step L next to R (8)

Restart

I Can't Help Myself (Sugar Pie, Honey Bunch) by Four Tops

SP, 32 count, 4 wall, right lead
Start at vocals, 24 beats into music

VINE RIGHT, SCUFF
STEP, SCUFF, STEP, SCUFF

1-4	Step R to right (1), step L behind R (2), step R to right (3), scuff L (4)
5-8	Step L (5), scuff R (6), step R (7), scuff L (8)

LINDY LEFT
PADDLE 1/8 LEFT X 2

1&2, 3-4	Triple step L (1), R (&), L (2) to left, rock R back (3), recover L (4)
5-6	Step R forward (5), paddle 1/8 turn L (6)
7-8	Step R forward (7), paddle 1/8 turn L (9:00) (8)

MONTANA KICK X 2

1-4	Step R forward (1), kick L forward (2), step L back (3), touch R back (4)
5-8	Step R forward (5), kick L forward (6), step L back (7), touch R back (8)

ROCKING CHAIR BACK X 2

1-4	Rock R back (1), step L in place (2), rock R forward (3), step L in place (4)
5-8	Rock R back (5), step L in place (6), rock R forward (7), step L in place (8)

Restart

I Do, I Do, I Do, I Do by ABBA
SP, 32 count, 2 wall, right lead
Start at vocals

STEP, CROSS POINT X 4

1-2	Step R to right (1), point L across R (2)
3-4	Step L to left (3), point R across L (4)
5-6	Step R to right (5), point L across R (6)
7-8	Step L to left (7), point R across L (8)

BASIC RIGHT, HITCH
BASIC LEFT, HITCH

1-4	Step R to right (1), step L together (2), step R to right (3), hitch L knee up (4)
5-8	Step L to left (5), step R together (6), step L to left (7), hitch R knee up (8)

PADDLE 1/4 LEFT X 2
BASIC RIGHT WITH TRIPLE TO RIGHT

1-2	Step R forward (1), paddle L with 1/4 turn left (9:00) (2)
3-4	Step R forward (3), paddle L with 1/4 turn left (6:00) (4)
5-6, 7&8	Step R to right (5), step L together (6), triple step R (7), L (&), R to right (8)

LINDY LEFT, SWAY RIGHT, LEFT, RIGHT, LEFT

1&2, 3-4	Triple step L (1), R (&), L (2) to left, rock R back (3), recover L (4)
5-8	Sway R (5), L (6), R (7), L (8)

Restart

(I Don't Know Why) But I Do
by Clarence "Frogman" Henry
KR, 32 count, 4 wall, right lead
Start at vocals "I don't know why…"

STEP, KICK X 4
1-2   Step R (1), kick L (2)
3-4   Step L (3), kick R (4)
5-6   Step R (5), kick L (6)
7-8   Step L (7), kick R (8)

LINDY RIGHT, LINDY LEFT
1&2, 3-4   Triple step R (1), L (&), R (2) to right,
                rock L behind R (3), recover R (4)
5&6, 7-8   Triple step L (5), R (&), L to left (6),
                rock R behind L (7), recover L (8)

ROCKING CHAIR WITH 1/4 TURN LEFT X 2
1-4   Rock R forward (1), step L in place (2), rock R back
        making 1/4 turn left (9:00) (3), step L in place (4)

5-8   Rock R forward (5), step L in place (6), rock R back
        making 1/4 turn left (6:00) (7), step L in place (8)

TRIPLE FORWARD X 2
JAZZ BOX WITH 1/4 TURN RIGHT
1&2   Triple step R (1), L (&), R (2) forward
3&4   Triple step L (3), R (&), L (4) forward

5-8   Step R across L (5), step L back (6),
        step R to right making 1/4 turn right (9:00) (7),
        step L next to R (8)

Restart

I'm Looking over a Four Leaf Clover by Mitch Miller
KR, 16 count, 4 wall, right lead
Start at vocals "I'm looking over…"

CHARLESTON

1-4	Touch R toe forward (1), step R next to L (2), touch L toe back (3), step L next to R (4)

HEEL, HEEL, BEHIND-SIDE-CROSS X 2

5-6	Touch R heel to right (5), touch R heel to right (6)
7&8	Step R behind L (7), step L to left (&), cross R over L (8)

1-2	Touch L heel to left (1), touch L heel to left (2)
3&4	Step L behind R (3), step R to right (&), cross L over R (4)

MONTEREY 1/4 TURN RIGHT

5-6	Point R to right (5), step R forward making 1/4 turn right (3:00) (6)
7-8	Point L to left (7), step L next to R (8)

Restart

Option: Replace Monterey turn with 2 pivots 1/8 L:
5-6	Step R forward (5), pivot 1/8 L (6)
7-8	Step R forward (7), pivot 1/8 L (9:00) (8)

I'm so Lonesome I Could Cry by Hank Williams

KR, 24 count, 2 wall, left lead, *waltz*
Begin on vocals "Hear that lonesome whippoorwill..."

MAMBO LEFT, MAMBO RIGHT

1-3   Rock L to left (1), recover R (2), step L next to R (3)
4-6   Rock R to right (4), recover L (5), step R next to L (6)

WALTZ FORWARD, WALTZ BACK WITH 1/4 TURN LEFT

1-3   Long step L forward (1), step R together (2),
           step L in place (3)
4-6   Long step R back making 1/4 turn left (9:00) (4),
           step L together (5), step R in place (6)

WALTZ FORWARD, WALTZ BACK WITH 1/4 TURN LEFT

1-3   Long step L forward (1), step R together (2),
           step L in place (3)
4-6   Long step R back making 1/4 turn left (6:00) (4),
           step L together (5), step R in place (6)

HESITATION FORWARD, HESITATION BACK

1-3   Long step L forward (1), step R together (2),
           hold going up on toes (3)

4-6   Long step R back (4), step L together (2)
           hold going up on toes (3)

Restart

In Search of Mona Lisa by Santana
KR, 32 count, 4 wall, right lead
Start 32 beats in, at vocals "Paris museum…"

POINT, STEP ACROSS X 4
1-2   Point R to right (1), step R across L (2)
3-4   Point L to left (3), step L across R (4)
5-6   Point R to right (5), step R across L (6)
7-8   Point L to left (7), step L across R (8)

MOON WALK 4 BACK
1   Slide R toe back, then heel down (1)
2   Slide L toe back, then heel down (2)
3   Slide R toe back, then heel down (3)
4   Slide L toe back, then heel down (4)

TRIPLE IN PLACE, ROCKING CHAIR
TRIPLE IN PLACE, ROCKING CHAIR
5&6   Triple R (5), L (&), R (6) in place
7-8, 1-2   Rock L forward (7), step R in place (8),
           rock L back (1), step R in place (2)

3&4   Triple L (3), R (&), L (4) in place
5-8   Rock R forward (5), step L in place (6),
       rock R back (7), step L in place (8)

PIVOT 1/4 LEFT X 2
JAZZ BOX WITH 1/4 TURN RIGHT
1-2   Step R forward (1), pivot 1/4 L (9:00) (2)
3-4   Step R forward (3), pivot 1/4 L (6:00) (4)

5-8   Step R across L (5), step L back (6),
       step R to right turning 1/4 right (9:00) (7),
       step L next to R (8)

Restart

In the Garden by Alan Jackson

KR, 24 count, 4 wall, left lead, *waltz*
Start at vocals "...come to the garden alone..."

LEFT TWINKLE, RIGHT TWINKLE WITH 1/4 TURN RIGHT

1-3	Cross step L over R (1), step R to right (2), step L slightly back behind R (3)
4-6	Cross step R over L (4), step L to left (5), step R slightly back while making 1/4 turn right (3:00)(6)

WALTZ LEFT FORWARD
WALTZ RIGHT BACK WITH 1/4 TURN LEFT

1-3	Long step L forward (1), step R next to L (2), step L in place (3)
4-6	Long step R back making 1/4 turn left (12:00) (4), step L next to R (5), step R in place (6)

HESITATION STEPS LEFT FORWARD, RIGHT BACK

1-3	Long step L forward(1), step R next to L (2), hold (going up on toes) (3)
4-6	Long step R back (4), step L next to R (5), hold (going up on toes) (3)

WALTZ LEFT BACK
WALTZ RIGHT FORWARD WITH 1/4 TURN RIGHT

1-3	Long step back L (1), step R next to L (2), step L in place (3)
4-6	Long step forward R while making 1/4 turn right (3:00) (4), step L next to R (5), step R in place (6)

Restart

In the Mood by Glenn Miller
SP, 16 count, 2 wall, right lead
Start after bugles, with melody

HEEL, HEEL, BEHIND-SIDE-CROSS X 2

1-2	Touch R heel to right (1), touch R heel to right (2)
3&4	Step R behind L (3), step L to left (&), cross R over L (4)

5-6	Touch L heel to left (5), touch L heel to left (6)
7&8	Step L behind R (7), step R to right (&), cross L over R (8)

FAST ROCKING CHAIR
PADDLE 1/4 LEFT

1&2&	Rock R forward (1), step L in place (&), rock R back (2), step L in place (&)
3-4	Step R forward (3), paddle 1/4 L (9:00) (4)

TRIPLE IN PLACE X 2

5&6	Triple R (5), L (&), R (6) in place
7&8	Triple L (7), R (&), L (8) in place

Restart

Inishannon Serenade by Frank Chacksfield
KR, 32 count, 2 wall, right lead
Start 16 beats in when music ratchets up a notch

STEP, DRAG X 2
RHUMBA RIGHT WITH TRIPLE BACK
1-2   Step R to right (1), drag L next to R (2)
3-4   Step L to left (3), drag R next to L (4)

5-6   Step R to right (5), step L together (6)
7&8   Triple step R (7), L (&), R back (8)

STEP, DRAG X 2
RHUMBA LEFT WITH TRIPLE FORWARD
1-2   Step L to left (1), drag R next to L (2)
3-4   Step R to right (3), drag L next to R (4)

5-6   Step L to left (5), step R together (6),
7&8   Triple step L (7), R (&), L (8) forward

ROCK RIGHT, RECOVER, CROSS TRIPLE TO LEFT
ROCK LEFT, RECOVER, CROSS TRIPLE TO RIGHT
1-2   Rock R to right (1), recover L (2)
3&4   Triple step R across L (3), L (&), R across L (4)
5-6   Rock L to left (5), recover R (6)
7&8   Triple step L across R (7), R (&), L across R (8)

TRIPLE WITH 1/8 TURN LEFT X 2
PIVOT 1/8 LEFT X 2

1&2   Triple step R (1), L (&), R (2) with 1/8 turn left
3&4   Triple step L (3), R (&), L (4) with 1/8 turn left (9:00)
5-6   Step R forward (5), pivot 1/8 L (6)
7-8   Step R forward (7), pivot 1/8 L (6:00) (8)

Restart

Tag: After wall 4: step, drag X 4.

Islands in the Stream by Dolly Parton and Kenny Rogers

SP, 32 count, 4 wall, right lead
Start 16 beats into music

V-STEP, TRIPLE RIGHT, TRIPLE LEFT

1-2	Step R to forward right (1), step L to forward left (2)
3-4	Step R back to center (3), step L next to R (4)
5&6	Triple step R (5), L (&), R (6) to right
7&8	Triple step L (7), R (&), L (8) to left

PADDLE 1/8 LEFT X 2
TRIPLE RIGHT, TRIPLE LEFT

1-2	Step R forward (1), paddle L with 1/8 left turn (2)
3-4	Step R forward (3), paddle L with 1/8 left turn (9:00) (4)
5&6	Triple step R (5), L (&), R (6) to right
7&8	Triple step L (7), R (&), L (8) to left

K-STEP WITH CLAPS

1-2	Step R to right forward diagonal (1), touch L next to R and clap (2)
3-4	Step L to left back diagonal (3), touch R next to L and clap (4)
5-6	Step R to right back diagonal (5), touch L next to R and clap (6)
7-8	Step L to left forward diagonal (7), touch R next to L and clap (8)

LINDY RIGHT, LINDY LEFT

1&2,3-4	Triple step R (1), L (&), R (2) to right, rock L back (3), recover R (4)
5&6,7-8	Triple step L (5), R (&), L (6) to left, rock R back (7), recover L (8)

Restart

Wall 5: Restart after paddle turns.

It Had to Be You by John Stevens
KR, 32 count, 4 wall, right lead
Start at vocals "...had to be you..."

WALK 3 FORWARD, KICK
WALK 3 BACK, KICK

1-4   Step R (1), L (2), R (3) forward, kick L across R (4)
5-8   Step L (5), R (6), L (7) back, kick R across L (8)

STEP, TOUCH X 2
BASIC RIGHT, TOUCH

1-2   Step R to right (1), touch L (2)
3-4   Step L to left (3), touch R (4)

5-8   Step R to right (5), step L together (6),
        step R to right (7), touch L next to R (8)

STEP, TOUCH X 2
LINDY LEFT WITH 1/4 TURN RIGHT

1-2   Step L to left (1), touch R (2)
3-4   Step R to right (3), touch L (4)

5&6, 7-8   Triple step L (5), R (&), L to left (6),
             rock R behind L making 1/4 turn right (3:00) (7),
             recover L (8)

ROCKING CHAIR
ROCK BACK, RECOVER X 2

1-4   Rock R forward (1), step L in place (2),
        rock R back (3), step L in place (4)
5-6   Rock R back (5), recover L (6)
7-8   Rock R back (7), recover L (8)

Restart

Karma Chameleon by Culture Club
KR, 16 count, 4 wall, right lead
Start after intro, with vocals

TRIPLE FORWARD X 2
MOON WALK 4 BACK

1&2	Triple R (1), L (&), R (2) forward
3&4	Triple L (3), R (&), L (4) forward

5	Slide R toe back, then heel down (5)
6	Slide L toe back, then heel down (6)
7	Slide R toe back, then heel down (7)
8	Slide L toe back, then heel down (8)

LINDY RIGHT
VINE LEFT WITH 1/4 TURN LEFT, TOUCH

1&2, 3-4   Triple step R (1), L (&), R (2) to right,
             rock L behind R (3), recover R (4)

5-8   Step L to left (5), step R behind L (6), step L to left
        making 1/4 turn left (9:00) (7), touch R next to L (8)

Restart

Love Train by The O Jays
KR, 32 count, 4 wall, right lead
Start 16 beats in at vocals

STEP, SCUFF FORWARD X 4

1-2	Step R (1), scuff L (2)
3-4	Step L (3), scuff R (4)
5-6	Step R (5), scuff L (6)
7-8	Step L (7), scuff R (8)

WALK 3 BACK, HITCH
X 2

1-4	Walk R (1), L (2), R (3) back, hitch L knee up (4)
5-8	Walk L (5), R (6), L (7) back, hitch R knee up (8)

TRIPLE TO RIGHT
1/2 TURN RIGHT AND TRIPLE TO LEFT
ROCKING CHAIR BACK

1&2	Triple R (1), L (&), R (2) to right
3&4	1/2 turn right and triple L (3), R (&), L (4) to left
5-8	Rock R back (5), step L in place (6), rock R forward (7), step L in place (8)

TRIPLE TO RIGHT
1/4 TURN RIGHT AND TRIPLE TO LEFT
ROCKING CHAIR BACK

1&2	Triple R (1), L (&), R (2) to right
3&4	1/4 turn right and triple L (3), R (&), L (4) to left
5-8	Rock R back (5), step L in place (6), rock R forward (7), step L in place (8)

Restart

Mambo Italiano by Bette Midler
SP, 16 count, 4 wall, right lead
Start at vocals "...Hey, mambo..."

MAMBO FORWARD, MAMBO BACK

1&2   Rock R forward (1), recover L back (&),
       step R next to L (2)
3&4   Rock L back (3), recover R (&),
       step L next to R (4)

SIDE ROCK RIGHT, RECOVER,
CROSS ROCK, RECOVER
X 2

5&6&7&8&   Rock R to right (5), recover L (&),
            rock R across L (6), recover L (&),
            rock R to right (7), recover L (&),
            rock R across L (8), recover L (&)

RHUMBA RIGHT FORWARD
RHUMBA LEFT BACK

1&2   Step R to right (1), step L next to R (&), step R forward (2)
3&4   Step L to left (3), step R next to L (&), step L back (4)

MAMBO BACK, HITCH AND TURN 1/4 LEFT
MAMBO BACK

5&6&   Rock R back (5), recover L (&),
       step R next to L (6), hitch L with 1/4 turn left (9:00) (&)
7&8   Rock L back (7), recover R (&), step L (8)

Restart

Option: ROCK, RECOVERS WITH TRAVEL:
Step slightly to left with each cross rock and each recover, to
travel left across the floor.

Midnight Train to Georgia
by Gladys Knight & The Pips
SP, 32 count, 4 wall, right lead
Start 16 beats after drum roll

VINE RIGHT, CROSS HEEL
STEP, CROSS HEEL, STEP, CROSS HEEL

1-4	Step R to right (1), step L behind R (2), step R to right (3), cross L heel over R (4)
5-6	Step L (5), cross R heel over L (6)
7-8	Step R (7), cross L heel over R (8)

VINE LEFT, CROSS HEEL
STEP, CROSS HEEL, STEP, CROSS HEEL

1-4	Step L to left (1), step R behind left (2), step L to left (3), cross R heel over L (4)
5-6	Step R (5), cross L heel over R (6)
7-8	Step L (7), cross R heel over L (8)

TRIPLE IN PLACE X 2
PADDLE 1/4 LEFT X 2

1&2	Triple step R (1), L (&), R (2) in place
3&4	Triple step L (3), R (&), L (4) in place
5-6	Step R forward (5), paddle L with 1/4 turn left (9:00) (6)
7-8	Step R forward (7), paddle L with 1/4 turn left (6:00) (8)

TRIPLE IN PLACE X 2
JAZZ BOX WITH 1/4 TURN RIGHT

1&2	Triple step R (1), L (&), R (2) in place
3&4	Triple step L (3), R (&), L (4) in place
5-8	Step R across L (5), step L back (6), step R to right turning 1/4 right (9:00) (7), step L next to R (8)

Restart

Mockingbird by Carly Simon and James Taylor

KR, 32 count, 4 wall, right lead
Start 20 beats in at vocals "Everybody, have you heard…"

STEP, SCUFF FORWARD X 4
1-2   Step R (1), scuff L (2)
3-4   Step L (3), scuff R (4)
5-6   Step R (5), scuff L (6)
7-8   Step L (7), scuff R (8)

WALK 3 BACK, HITCH
WALK 3 BACK, HITCH
1-4   Step R (1), L (2), R (3) back,
          hitch L knee up with a little kick (4)

5-8   Step L (5), R (6), L (7) back,
          hitch R knee up with a little kick (8)

BASIC RIGHT, FLAT LEFT
FAN LEFT, FRONT, LEFT, FRONT
1-4   Step R to right (1), step L together (2), step R to right (3),
          touch flat L (4)

5-8   Fan L toe to left (5), then front (6), then left (7),
          then front (8)

LINDY LEFT WITH 1/4 TURN RIGHT
1&2, 3-4   Triple step L (1), R (&), L to left (2),
                rock R behind L making 1/4 turn right (3:00) (3),
                recover L (4)

ROCK BACK, RECOVER X 2
5-6   Rock R back (5), recover L (6)
7-8   Rock R back (7), recover L (8)

Restart

Option: Replace rock back, recover with kick-ball-change:
5&6   Kick R forward (5),
          step on ball of R while raising L (&), step L (6)
7&8   Kick R foot forward (7),
          step on ball of R while raising L (&), step L (8)

Molly Malone by The Dubliners
KR, 24 count, 1 wall, left lead, *waltz*
Begin after 24 beats on vocals "...Dublin's fair city..."

WALTZ FORWARD
WALTZ BACK WITH 1/4 TURN LEFT

1-3   Long step L forward (1), step R together (2),
             step L in place (3)
4-6   Long step R back making 1/4 turn left (9:00) (4),
             step L together (5), step R in place (6)

LEFT TWINKLE, RIGHT TWINKLE

1-3   Step L across R (1), step R to right (2),
             step L slightly back behind R (3)
4-6   Step R across L (4), step L to left (5),
             step R slightly back behind L (6)

LEFT TWINKLE, RIGHT TWINKLE WITH 1/4 TURN RIGHT

1-3   Step L across R (1), step R to right (2),
             step L slightly back behind R (3)
4-6   Step R across L (4), step L to left (5),
             step R slightly back making 1/4 turn right (12:00) (6)

WALTZ FORWARD
WALTZ BACK WITH 1/4 TURN LEFT

1-3   Long step L forward (1), step R together (2),
             step L in place (3)
4-6   Long step R back making 1/4 turn left (9:00) (4),
             step L together (5), step R in place (6)

Restart

Mr. Sandman by The Chordettes
SP, 32 count, 4 wall, right lead
Start 16 beats into music

STEP, SLIDE X 4

1-2	Step R to right (1), slide L next to R (2)
3-4	Step L to left (3), slide R next to L (4)
5-6	Step R to right (5), slide L next to R (6)
7-8	Step L to left (7), slide R next to L (8)

ROCKING CHAIR
V-STEP

1-4   Rock R forward (1), step L in place (2),
       rock R back (3), step L in place (4)
5-6   Step R to forward right (5), step L to forward left (6)
7-8   Step R back to center (7), step L next to R (8)

VINE RIGHT, KICK ACROSS
VINE LEFT, KICK ACROSS

1-4   Step R to right (1), step L behind R (2),
       step R to right (3), kick L across R (4)

5-8   Step L to left (5), step R behind L (6),
       step L to left (7), kick R across L (8)

V-STEP
HEEL BOUNCE 4 WITH 1/4 TURN LEFT

1-2   Step R to forward right (1), step L to forward left (2)
3-4   Step R back to center (3), step L next to R (4)
5-8   Heel bounce (5), (6), (7), (8)
       making 1/4 turn left (9:00)

Restart

My Girl by The Temptations
SP, 32 count, 4 wall, right lead
Start at vocals, 16 beats into music

BASIC RIGHT, TRIPLE TO RIGHT
LINDY LEFT

1-2, 3&4	Step R to right (1), step L together (2), triple step R (3), L (&), R (4) to right
5&6, 7-8	Triple step L (5), R (&), L (6) to left, rock R behind L (7), recover L (8)

BASIC RIGHT, TRIPLE TO RIGHT
LINDY LEFT

1-2, 3&4	Step R to right (1), step L together (2), triple step R (3), L (&), R (4) to right
5&6, 7-8	Triple step L (5), R (&), L (6) to left, rock R behind L (7), recover L (8)

PADDLE 1/8 LEFT X 2

1-2	Step R (1), paddle L with 1/4 turn left (2)
3-4	Step R (3), paddle L with 1/4 turn left (9:00) (4)

SHUFFLE BOX RIGHT FORWARD, LEFT BACK

5-6, 7&8	Step R to right (5), step L together (6), triple step R (7), L (&), R (8) forward
1-2, 3&4	Step L to left (1), step R together (2), triple step L (3), R (&), L (4) back

ROCKING CHAIR BACK

5-8	Rock R back (5), step L in place (6), rock R forward (7), step L in place (8)

Restart

No No Song by Ringo Starr
KR, 32 count, 4 wall, right lead
Start at vocals "A lady that I know…"

TOE STRUT FORWARD
X 4

1-2	Step R toe forward (1), come down on R heel (2)
3-4	Step L toe forward (3), come down on L heel (4)
5-6	Step R toe forward (5), come down on R heel (6)
7-8	Step L toe forward (7), come down on L heel (8)

WALK 3 BACK, HITCH
WALK 3 BACK, HITCH

1-4	Step R (1), L (2), R (3) back, hitch L knee up with a little kick (4)
5-8	Step L (5), R (6), L (7) back, hitch R knee up with a little kick (8)

LINDY RIGHT
LINDY LEFT WITH 1/4 TURN RIGHT

1&2, 3-4	Triple step R (1), L (&), R (2) to right, rock L behind R (3), recover R (4)
5&6, 7-8	Triple step L (5), R (&), L to left (6), rock R behind L making 1/4 turn right (3:00) (7), recover L (8)

ROCKING CHAIR
X 2

1-4	Rock R forward R (1), step L in place (2), rock R back (3), step L in place (4)
5-8	Rock R forward (5), step L in place (6), rock R back (7), step L in place (8)

Restart

Tag: After walls 2 and 5, add 2 toe struts.

Poor Little Fool by Ricky Nelson
SP, 32 count, 2 wall, right lead
Start at vocals

STEP FORWARD, POINT FORWARD, COASTER
X 2

1-2	Step R forward (1), point L forward (2)
3&4	Step L back (3), step R next to L (&), step L (4)
5-6	Step R forward (5), touch forward L (6)
7&8	Step L back (7), step R next to L (&), step L (8)

WALK 3 FORWARD, POINT FORWARD
WALK 2 BACK, COASTER

1-4	Walk R (1), L (2), R (3) forward, point L forward (4)
5-6	Walk L (5), R (6) back
7&8	Step L back (7), step R next to L (&), step L (8)

PADDLE 1/4 LEFT X 2

1-2	Step R forward (1), paddle L with 1/4 turn left (9:00) (2)
3-4	Step R forward (3), paddle L with 1/4 turn left (6:00) (4)

LINDY RIGHT
LINDY LEFT

5&6, 7-8	Triple step R (5), L (&), R (6) to right, rock L back (7), recover R (8)
1&2, 3-4	Triple step L (1), R (&), L (2) to left, rock R back (3), recover L (4)

V-STEP

5-6	Step R to forward right (5), step L to forward left (6)
7-8	Step R back to center (7), step L next to R (8)

Restart

Ready to Roll by Blake Shelton
SP, 16 count, 4 wall, right lead
Start at vocals, 24 beats into music

TOUCH RIGHT OUT, IN, COASTER

1-2   Touch R out to right (1), in (2)
3&4   Step R back (3), step L next to R (&), step R forward (4)

TOUCH LEFT OUT, IN, COASTER

5-6   Touch L out to left (5), in (6)
7&8   Step L back (7), step R next to L (&), step L forward (8)

TRIPLE FORWARD X 2
PADDLE 1/8 LEFT X 2

1&2   Triple R (1), L (&), R (2) forward
3&4   Triple L (3), R (&), L (4) forward
5-6   Step R forward (5), paddle 1/8 turn L (6)
7-8   Step R forward (7), paddle 1/8 turn L (9:00) (8)

Restart

Release Me by The Mills Brothers
KR, 32 count, 4 wall, right lead
Start at vocals "Please release me…"

STEP, POINT
X 4

1-2	Step R forward (1), point L to left (2)
3-4	Step L across R (3), point R to right (4)
5-6	Step R across L (5), point L to left (6)
7-8	Step L across R (7), point R to right (8)

BACK, BACK, TRIPLE BACK
X 2

1-2	Step R back (1), L back (2)
3&4	Triple R (3), L (&), R (4) back
5-6	Step L back (5), R back (6)
7&8	Triple L (7), R (&), L (8) back

MONTEREY 1/4 TURN RIGHT
X 2

1-2	Point R to right (1), step R forward making 1/4 turn right (3:00) (2)
3-4	Point L to left (3), step L next to R (4)
5-6	Point R to right (5), step R forward making 1/4 turn right (6:00) (6)
7-8	Point L to left (7), step L next to R (8)

LINDY RIGHT, LINDY LEFT WITH 1/4 TURN RIGHT

1&2, 3-4	Triple step R (1), L (&), R (2) to right, rock L back (3), recover R (4)
5&6, 7-8	Triple step L (5), R (&), L to left (6), rock R behind L making 1/4 turn right (9:00) (7), recover L (8)

Restart

Seven Year Ache by Rosanne Cash
KR, 32 count, 2 wall, right lead
Start at vocals "You act like you were just born tonight…"

LOCK STEPS FORWARD RIGHT, TOUCH
LOCK STEPS FORWARD LEFT, TOUCH

1-4   Step R diagonally forward to right (1), lock L behind R (2),
          step R diagonally forward to right (3), touch L next to R (4)
5-8   Step L diagonally forward to left (5), lock R behind L (6),
          step L diagonally forward to left (7), touch R next to L (8)

WALK 3 BACK, HITCH
X 2

1-4   Step R back (1), L back (2), R back (3),
          hitch L knee up with a little kick (4)
5-8   Step L back (5), R back (6), L back (7),
          hitch R knee up with a little kick (8)

SWAY, TOUCH
X 4

1-2   Sway R (1), touch L next to R (2)
3-4   Sway L (3), touch R next to L (4)
5-6   Sway R (5), touch L next to R (6)
7-8   Sway L (7), touch R next to L (8)

TRIPLE WITH 1/8 TURN LEFT X 2
PIVOT 1/8 LEFT X 2

1&2   Triple step R (1), L (&), R (2) with 1/8 turn left
3&4   Triple step L (3), R (&), L (4) with 1/8 turn left (9:00)
5-6   Step R forward (5), pivot 1/8 L (6)
7-8   Step R forward (7), pivot 1/8 L (6:00) (8)

Restart

Silhouettes by the Rays
SP, 32 count, 4 wall, right lead
Start 16 beats into music

TRIPLE TO RIGHT, TRIPLE TO LEFT
V-STEP

1&2   Triple step R (1), L (&), R (2) to right
3&4   Triple step L (3), R (&), L (4) to left
5-6   Step R to forward right (5), step L to forward left (6)
7-8   Step R back to center (7), step L next to R (8)

TRIPLE TO RIGHT, TRIPLE TO LEFT
PADDLE 1/4 LEFT X 2

1&2   Triple step R (1), L (&), R (2) to right
3&4   Triple step L (3), R (&), L (4) to left
5-6   Step R (5), paddle L with 1/4 turn left (9:00)(6)
7-8   Step R (7), paddle L with 1/4 turn left (6:00) (8)

ROCK RIGHT, RECOVER, COASTER
ROCK LEFT, RECOVER, COASTER

1-2   Rock R to right (1), recover L (2),
3&4   Step R back (3), step L next to R (&), step R (4)
5-6   Rock L to left (5), recover R (6)
7&8   Step L back (7), step R next to L (&), step L (8)

SAILOR RIGHT, SAILOR LEFT

1&2   Step R behind L (1), step L to left (&),
       step R to right (2)
3&4   Step L behind R (3), step R to right (&),
       step L to left (4)

SAILOR RIGHT WITH 1/4 TURN RIGHT, STEP, TOUCH

5&6   Step R behind L with 1/4 turn right (9:00) (5),
       step L to left (&), step R to right (6)
7-8   Step L (7), touch R (8)

Restart

Sixteen Candles by The Crests
SP, 32 count, 2 wall, right lead
Start at vocals "...candles..."

ROCK FORWARD, RECOVER, TRIPLE BACK
ROCK BACK, RECOVER, TRIPLE FORWARD

1-2, 3&4	Rock R forward (1), recover L back (2), triple step R (3), L (&), R (4) back
5-6,7&8	Rock L back (5), recover R (6), triple step L (7), R (&), L (8) forward

ROCK RIGHT, RECOVER, CROSS TRIPLE
ROCK LEFT, RECOVER, CROSS TRIPLE

1-2, 3&4	Rock R to right (1), recover L (2), triple step R across L (3), L (&), R across L (4)
5-6, 7&8	Rock L to left (5), recover R (6) triple step L across R (7), R (&), L across R (8)

K-STEP SHUFFLE:
RIGHT DIAGONAL FORWARD, TOUCH, TRIPLE HOME
RIGHT DIAGONAL BACK, TOUCH, TRIPLE HOME

1-2	Step R diagonal forward (1), touch L next to R (2)
3&4	Triple step L (3), R (&), L (4) diagonally left back to home
5-6	Step R diagonal back (5), touch L next to R (6)
7&8	Triple step L (7), R (&), L (8) diagonally forward to home

CROSS STEP RIGHT, POINT LEFT
CROSS STEP LEFT, POINT RIGHT
PADDLE 1/4 LEFT X 2

1-2	Step R across L (1), point L to left (2)
3-4	Step L across R (3), point R to right (4)
5-6	Step forward R (5), paddle L with 1/4 turn left (9:00) (6)
7-8	Step forward R (7), paddle L with 1/4 turn left (6:00) (8)

Restart

Soldier Boy by The Shirelles
SP, 32 count, 4 wall, right lead
Start 32 beats into music

LINDY RIGHT, LINDY LEFT

1&2,3-4	Triple step R (1), L (&), R (2) to right, rock L back (3), recover R (4)
5&6,7-8	Triple step L (5), R (&), L (6) to left, rock R back (7), recover L (8)

VINE RIGHT, CROSS
SIDE ROCK, RECOVER, CROSS TRIPLE

1-4	Step R to right (1), step L behind R (2), step R to right (3), cross L over R (4)
5-6, 7&8	Rock R to right (5), recover L (6), cross triple R (7), L (&), R (8) to left

VINE LEFT, CROSS
SIDE ROCK, RECOVER, CROSS TRIPLE

1-4	Step L to left (1), step R behind L (2), step L to left (3), cross R over L (4)
5-6, 7&8	Rock L to left (5), recover R (6), cross triple L (7), R (&), L (8) to right

PADDLE 1/8 LEFT X 2
STEP, TOUCH X 2

1-2	Step R forward (1), paddle L with 1/8 turn left (2)
3-4	Step R forward (3), paddle L with 1/8 turn left (9:00) (4)
5-6	Step R (5), touch L next to R (6)
7-8	Step L (7), touch R next to L (8)

Restart

Something's Gotta Give by The McGuire Sisters
KR, 32 count, 2 wall, right lead
Start at vocals "When an irresistible force such as you..."

RHUMBA RIGHT BACK, HOLD
RHUMBA LEFT FORWARD, HOLD
1-4   Step R to right (1), step L together (2),
        step R back (3), hold (4)
5-8   Step L to left (5), step R together (6),
        step L forward (7), hold (8)

RHUMBA RIGHT BACK, HOLD
RHUMBA LEFT FORWARD, HOLD
1-4   Step R to right (1), step L together (2),
        step R back (3), hold (4)
5-8   Step L to left (5), step R together (6),
        step L forward (7), hold (8)

ROCKING CHAIR X 2
1-4   Rock R forward (1), step L in place (2),
        rock R back (3), step L in place (4)
5-8   Rock R forward (5), step L in place (6),
        rock R back (7), step L in place (8)

SLOW PIVOT 1/4 LEFT X 2
1-4   Step R forward (1-2), pivot 1/4 L (9:00) (3-4)
5-8   Step R forward (5-6), pivot 1/4 L (6:00) (7-8)

Restart

Option: Replace 2 slow pivots with:
A - 4 pivots 1/8 L, or
B - 2 step, points and 2 pivots 1/4 L:
    1-2 Step R forward (1), point L to side (2)
    3-4 Step L forward(3), point R to side (4)
    5-6 Step R forward (5), pivot 1/4 L (9:00) (6)
    7-8 Step R forward (7), pivot 1/4 L (6:00) (8)

Soul Man by Sam & Dave
SP, 32 count, 4 wall, right lead
Start 32 beats in, at vocals

STEP RIGHT, TOGETHER, TRIPLE TO RIGHT
LINDY LEFT

1-2, 3&4	Step R (1), L together (2), triple R (3), L (&), R (4) to right
5&6,7-8	Triple step L (5), R (&), L (6) to left, rock R back (7), recover L (8)

STEP RIGHT, TOGETHER, TRIPLE TO RIGHT
LINDY LEFT

1-2, 3&4	Step R (1), L together (2), triple R (3), L (&), R (4) to right
5&6,7-8	Triple step L (5), R (&), L (6) to left, rock R back (7), recover L (8)

RHUMBA RIGHT FORWARD, TOUCH
RHUMBA LEFT BACK, TOUCH

1-4	Step R to right (1), step L together (2) step R forward (3), touch L next to R (4)
5-8	Step L to left (5), step R together (6), step L back (7), touch R next to L (8)

STEP, TOUCH X 2
JAZZ BOX WITH 1/4 TURN RIGHT

1-2	Step R (1), touch L (2)
3-4	Step L (3), touch R (4)
5-8	Step R across L (5), step L back (6), step R to right making 1/4 turn right (3:00) (7), step L next to R (8)

Restart

Swingin' by John Anderson
KR, 32 count, 4 wall, right lead
Start at vocals "There's a little girl, in our neighborhood…"

STEP, LOCK, TRIPLE FORWARD RIGHT
STEP, LOCK, TRIPLE FORWARD LEFT
1-2, 3&4   Step R forward right (1), lock L behind R (2),
              triple R (3), L (&), R (4) forward right
5-6, 7&8   Step L forward left (5), lock R behind L (6),
              triple L (7), R (&), L (8) forward left

WALK 4 BACK WITH 1/2 TURN LEFT
1-4   Step R (1), L (2), R (3), L (4) back,
        making 1/2 turn left (6:00)

JAZZ BOX WITH 1/4 TURN RIGHT
5-8   Step R across L (5), step L back (6),
        step R to right turning 1/4 right (9:00) (7),
        step L next to R (8)

TRIPLE RIGHT, TRIPLE LEFT
1&2   Triple step R (1), L (&), R (2) to right
3&4   Triple step L (3), R (&), L (4) to left

LINDY RIGHT, LINDY LEFT
5&6, 7-8   Triple step R (5), L (&), R (6) to right,
              rock L back (7), recover R (8)
1&2, 3-4   Triple step L (1), R (&), L (2) to left,
              rock R back (3), recover L (4)

ROCK BACK, RECOVER X 2
5-6   Rock R back (5), recover L (6)
7-8   Rock R back (7), recover L (8)

Restart

Take a Chance on Me by ABBA
SP, 16 count, 4 wall, right lead
Start at vocals "…if you're all alone…"

ROCKING CHAIR
PADDLE 1/8 LEFT X 2

1-4   Rock R forward (1), step L in place (2),
         rock R back (3), step L in place (4)

5-6   Step R forward (5), paddle L with 1/8 turn left (6)
7-8   Step R forward (7), paddle L with 1/8 turn left (9:00) (8)

BASIC RIGHT WITH TRIPLE
LINDY LEFT

1-2, 3&4   Step R to right (1), step L together (2),
         triple step R (3), L (&), R (4) to right

5&6, 7-8   Triple step L (5), R (&), L (6) to left,
         rock R back (7), recover L (8)

Restart

Tennessee Waltz by Patti Page
KR, 48 count, 2 wall, left lead, *waltz*
Start at vocals "I was dancin' with my darlin'…"

WALTZ BOX FORWARD, BACK X 2
1-3   Long step L forward (1), step R to forward right (2),
        step L together (3)
4-6   Long step R back (4), step L to back L (5),
        step R together (6)
1-3   Long step L forward (1), step R to forward right (2),
        step L together (3)
4-6   Long step R back (4), step L to back L (5),
        step R together (6)
TWINKLE, TWINKLE WITH 1/4 TURN RIGHT X 2
1-3   Step L across R (1), step R to right (2),
        step L slightly back behind R (3)
4-6   Step R across L (4), step L to left (5),
        step R slightly back making 1/4 turn right (3:00) (6)
1-3   Step L across R (1), step R to right (2),
        step L slightly back behind R (3)
4-6   Step R across L (4), step L to left (5),
        step R slightly back making 1/4 turn right (6:00) (6)
WALTZ FORWARD, WALTZ BACK WITH 1/4 TURN LEFT X 4
1-3   Long step L forward (1), step R together (2),
        step L in place (3)
4-6   Long step R back making 1/4 turn left (3:00) (4),
        step L together (5), step R in place (6)
1-3   Long step L forward (1), step R together (2),
        step L in place (3)
4-6   Long step R back making 1/4 turn left (12:00) (4),
        step L together (5), step R in place (6)
1-3   Long step L forward (1), step R together (2),
        step L in place (3)
4-6   Long step R back making 1/4 turn left (9:00) (4),
        step L together (5), step R in place (6)
1-3   Long step L forward (1), step R together (2),
        step L in place (3)
4-6   Long step R back making 1/4 turn left (6:00) (4),
        step L together (5), step R in place (6)

Restart

Tequila by The Champs
SP, 24 count, 4 wall, left lead
Begin when sax intones

SHUFFLE BOX LEFT FORWARD, RIGHT BACK

1-2, 3&4	Step L to left (1), step R together (2), triple L (3), R (&), L (4) forward
5-6, 7&8	Step R to right (5), step L together (6), triple R (7), L (&), R (8) back

HALF SHUFFLE BOX LEFT FORWARD
MAMBO RIGHT, MAMBO LEFT

1-2, 3&4	Step L to left (1), step R together (2), triple L (3), R (&), L (4) forward
5&6	Rock R to right (5), recover L (&), step R next to L (6)
7&8	Rock L to left (7), recover R (&), step L next to R (8)

MONTEREY 1/4 TURN RIGHT
ELVIS KNEES RIGHT, LEFT, RIGHT& RIGHT&

1-2	Point R to right (1), step R forward making 1/4 turn right (3:00) (2)
3-4	Point L to left (3), step L next to R (4)
5-6, 7&8&	With weight on balls of feet, pop R knee in (5), then L knee (6), R knee (7), L knee (&), R knee (8), L knee (&)

Restart

The Lion Sleeps Tonight (Wimoweh) by The Tokens
SP, 64 count, 2 wall, right lead
Start at vocals "In the jungle…"

STEP, TOUCH FORWARD X 4
1-2 Step R forward right (1), touch L next to R (2)
3-4 Step L forward left (3), touch R next to L (4)
5-6 Step R forward right (5), touch L next to R (6)
7-8 Step L forward left (7), touch R next to L (8)
K-STEP WITH CLAPS
1-2 Step R forward right (1), touch L next to R and clap (2)
3-4 Step L back left (3), touch R next to L and clap (4)
5-6 Step R back right (5), touch L next to R and clap (6)
7-8 Step L forward left (7), touch R next to L and clap (8)
STEP, TOUCH BACK X 4
1-2 Step R back right (1), touch L next to R (2)
3-4 Step L back left (3), touch R next to L (4)
5-6 Step R back right (5), touch L next to R (6)
7-8 Step L back left (7), touch R next to L (8)
K-STEP WITH CLAPS
1-2 Step R forward right (1), touch L next to R and clap (2)
3-4 Step L back left (3), touch R next to L and clap (4)
5-6 Step R back right (5), touch L next to R and clap (6)
7-8 Step L forward left (7), touch R next to L and clap (8)
RIGHT DIAGONAL FORWARD 3, KICK, BACK 3, TOUCH
1-4 Step R (1), L (2), R (3) diagonally forward to right, kick L (4)
5-8 Step L (5), R (6), L (7) back, touch R next to L (8)
LEFT DIAGONAL FORWARD 3, KICK, BACK 3, TOUCH
1-4 Step R (1), L (2), R (3) diagonally forward to left, kick L (4)
5-8 Step L (5), R (6), L (7) back, touch R next to L (8)
PADDLE 1/8 LEFT X 2
1-2 Step R forward (1), paddle L with 1/8 turn left (2)
3-4 Step R forward (3), paddle L with 1/8 turn left (9:00) (4)
MONTANA KICK X 2
5-8 Step R forward (5), kick L forward (6),
    step L back (7), touch R back (8)
1-4 Step R forward (1), kick L forward (2),
    step L back (3), touch R back (4)
PADDLE 1/8 LEFT X 2
5-6 Step R forward (5), paddle L with 1/8 turn left (6)
7-8 Step R forward (7), paddle L with 1/8 turn left (6:00) (8)

Restart

71

The Wanderer by Dion
SP, 32 count, 4 wall, right lead
Start 16 beats into music

VINE RIGHT, SCUFF
STEP, SCUFF, STEP, SCUFF

1-4	Step R to right (1), step L behind R (2), step R to right (3), scuff L (4)
5-8	Step L (5), scuff R (6), step R (7), scuff L (8)

K-STEP TO LEFT WITH CLAPS

1-2	Step L to forward left (1), touch R next to L and clap (2)
3-4	Step R to back right (3), touch L next to R and clap (4)
5-6	Step L to back left (5), touch R next to L and clap (6)
7-8	Step R to forward right (7), touch L next to R and clap (8)

VINE LEFT, SCUFF
STEP, SCUFF, STEP, SCUFF

1-4	Step L to left (1), step R behind L (2), step L to left (3), scuff R (4)
5-8	Step R (5), scuff L (6), step L (7), scuff R (8)

V-STEP
BOUNCE 4 WITH 1/4 TURN LEFT

1-2	Step R to forward right (1), step L to forward left (2)
3-4	Step R back to center (3), step L next to R (4)
5-8	Bounce (5), bounce (6), bounce (7), bounce (8) with weight on toes while making 1/4 turn left (9:00)

Restart

Uptown by Roy Orbison
SP, 32 count, 4 wall, right lead
Start 16 beats into music

RHUMBA RIGHT FORWARD, HOLD
RHUMBA LEFT FORWARD, HOLD

1-4   Step R to right (1), step L together (2),
       step R forward (3), hold (4)
5-8   Step L to left (5), step R together (6),
       step L forward (7), hold (8)

WALK 3 BACK, HITCH
X 2

1-4   Walk R (1), L (2), R (3) back, hitch L knee up (4)
5-8   Walk L (5), R (6), L (7) back, hitch R knee up (8)

TOUCH RIGHT OUT, IN, STEP, SLIDE
TOUCH LEFT OUT, IN, STEP, SLIDE

1-4   Touch R out to right (1), in (2), step R to right (3),
       slide L together (4)
5-8   Touch L out to left (5), in (6), step L to left (7),
       slide R together (8)

1/4 TURN LEFT AND TOUCH RIGHT OUT, IN, STEP, SLIDE
DIAGONAL STEPS FORWARD TO LEFT, SLIDE

1-4   Touch R out diagonally forward to right (1), in (2),
       step R diagonally forward to right (3), slide L together (4)
5-8   Step L (5), R (6), L (7) diagonally forward to left,
       slide R together and face 9 o'clock (9:00) (8)

Restart

Western Girls by Marty Stuart
SP, 32 count, 4 wall, right lead
Start 32 beats into music

SHIMMY RIGHT X 2

1-4	Step R to right (1-2), L together (3-4)
	while moving shoulders forward and back
5-8	Step R to right (5-6), L together (7-8)
	while moving shoulders forward and back

BASIC RIGHT, LEFT HEEL
BASIC LEFT, DOUBLE STOMP
FAN RIGHT OUT, IN, OUT, IN

1-4	Step R to side (1), step L together (2),
	step R to side (3), touch L heel down (4)
5-8&	Step L to side (5), step R together (6),
	step L to side (7), stomp R heel down (8),
	stomp R heel down (&)
1-4	Fan R out (1), in (2), out (3), in (4)

WALK 2 BACK, 1/4 TURN RIGHT, HITCH
WALK 3 BACK, DOUBLE STOMP
FAN RIGHT OUT, IN, OUT, IN

5-8	Step back R (5), L (6), 1/4 turn R (3:00) (7),
	hitch L knee up (8)
1-4&	Step back L (1), R (2), L (3), stomp R heel down (4),
	stomp R heel down (&)
5-8	Fan R out (5), in (6), out (7), in (8)

Restart

Y'all Come Back Saloon by The Oak Ridge Boys
KR, 32 count, 1 wall, right lead
Start after 8 beats at vocals "…tambourine with a silver jingle…"

ROCK FORWARD, BACK, TRIPLE BACK
ROCK BACK, FORWARD, TRIPLE FORWARD
1-2, 3&4   Rock R forward (1), recover L (2),
              triple R (3), L (&), R (4) back
5-6,7&8   Rock L back (5), recover R (6),
              triple L (7), R (&), L (8) forward

RIGHT FORWARD, 1/2 TURN LEFT, TRIPLE IN PLACE
LEFT FORWARD, 1/4 TURN RIGHT, TRIPLE IN PLACE
1-2, 3&4   Rock R forward (1), 1/2 turn L (6:00) (2),
              triple R (3), L (&), R (4) in place
5-6,7&8   Rock L forward (5), 1/2 turn R (9:00) (6),
              triple L (7), R (&), L (8) in place

LINDY RIGHT, LINDY LEFT
1&2, 3-4   Triple step R (1), L (&), R (2) to right,
              rock L back (3), recover R (4)
5&6, 7-8   Triple step L (5), R (&), L (6) to left,
              rock R back (7), recover L (8)

JAZZ BOX WITH 1/4 TURN RIGHT
STEP, TOUCH X 2
1-4   Step R across L (1), step L back (2),
       step R to right turning 1/4 right (12:00) (3),
       step L next to R (4)
5-6   Step R (5), touch L (6)
7-8   Step L (7), touch R (8)

Restart

Tag: After walls 1, 2 and 4: Step R, step L.

You're Nobody 'til Somebody Loves You by Dean Martin
KR, 32 count, 2 wall, right lead
Start at vocals "You're nobody 'til somebody..."

LOCK STEPS FORWARD RIGHT, TOUCH
LOCK STEPS FORWARD LEFT, TOUCH

1-4	Step R diagonally forward to right (1), lock L behind R (2), step R diagonally forward to right (3), touch L next to R (4)
5-8	Step L diagonally forward to left (5), lock R behind L (6), step L diagonally forward to left (7), touch R next to L (8)

STEP, TOUCH BACK DIAGONAL
X 4

1-2	Step R to back right (1), touch L next to R (2)
3-4	Step L to back left (3), touch R next to L (4)
5-6	Step R to back right (5), touch L next to R (6)
7-8	Step L to back left (7), touch R next to L (8)

VINE RIGHT, TOUCH
VINE LEFT, TOUCH

1-4	Step R to right (1), step L behind R (2), step R to right (3), touch L next to R (4)
5-8	Step L to left (5), step R behind left (6), step L to left (7), touch R next to left (8)

ROCKING CHAIR WITH 1/4 TURN LEFT
X 2

1-4	Rock R forward (1), step L in place (2), rock R back making 1/4 turn left (9:00) (3), step L in place (4)
5-8	Rock R forward (5), step L in place (6), rock R back making 1/4 turn left (12:00) (7), step L in place (8)

Restart

SONGS FOR THE DANCES

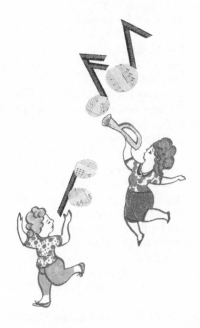

Each dance can be danced to multiple songs.

PLEASE NOTE: Tags and restarts listed in the step sheets are only for the numbered songs. Other songs should be danceable without tags, but may require restarts to stay with the music.

1 A Kiss to Build a Dream on by Louis Armstrong
Amor by Eydie Gorme and Los Panchos
December, 1963 (Oh What A Night)
by Frankie Valli & The Four Seasons
Have Yourself a Merry Little Christmas
by Vince Vance & The Valiants
Neon Moon by Brooks & Dunn
On and On by Stephen Bishop
Over the Rainbow by Israel Ka'ano'i Kamakawiwo'ole
Santa Baby by Eartha Kitt with Henri Rene & His Orchestra
True Love Ways by Mickey Gilley
Walkin' My Baby Back Home by Nat King Cole

2 Act Naturally by Buck Owens
Bad Moon Rising by Creedence Clearwater Revival
Christmas Cookies by George Strait
Fourteen Carat Mind by Gene Watson
I'll Sail My Ship Alone by Moon Mullican
If You Wanna Be Happy by Dr. Victor
Oh Lonesome Me by Don Gibson
Sea of Heartbreak by Don Gibson
The Same Way You Came In by Big Tom

3 Ain't That a Kick in the Head by Dean Martin
Come Softly To Me by The Fleetwoods
On the Sunny Side of the Street
by Tony Bennett and Willie Nelson
Red Sails in the Sunset by Johnny Lee
Singin' in the Rain by Doris Day
Sugar Shack by Jimmy Gilmer & The Fireballs
Why Don't We Just Dance by Josh Turner

4 Ain't Too Proud to Beg by The Temptations
1-2-3 by Len Barry
Alley Oop by Hollywood Argyles
Cathy's Clown by The Everly Brothers
I'll Never Find Another You by The Seekers
She's Not There by The Zombies
Stay by Maurice Williams & The Zodiacs

5 All I Do Is Dream of You by Michael Bublé
All of Me by Michael Buble
Fly Me to the Moon by Scooter Lee
Here Lately by Scooter Lee
Show Me the Way to Go Home by Jimmy and the Parrots

6 All My Exes Live in Texas by George Strait
Coal Miner's Daughter by Loretta Lynn
Garden Party by Ricky Nelson
Put Your Hand in the Hand by Ocean
Trashy Women by Confederate Railroad
Viva La Vida by Coldplay
Wagon Wheel by Darius Rucker
Working in the Coal Mine by Lee Dorsey
Your Mama Don't Dance by Loggins & Messina

7 Anything Goes by Frank Sinatra
Catch a Falling Star by Perry Como
I Can See Clearly Now by Johnny Nash
I'll Get Over You by Helen McCaffrey
Let Your Love Flow by The Bellamy Brothers
Love is Here to Stay by Frank Sinatra
On the Street Where You Live by Dean Martin
Personality by Lloyd Price
Red Roses for a Blue Lady by Johnny Tillotson
She's Not You by Luca Olivieri

8 (Baby) Hully Gully by The Olympics
A White Sport Coat (and A Pink Carnation) by Marty Robbins
Big Spender by Peggy Lee
I'll Be Around by The Spinners
I'm Gonna Get Married by Lloyd Price
Lady Luck by Lloyd Price
No If's – No And's by Lloyd Price
Only the Lonely by Roy Orbison
Santa Claus is Back in Town by Elvis Presley
Shotgun by Jr. Walker & The All Stars

9 Be My Baby by The Ronettes
Alley Cat by Chet Atkins
Come Monday by Jimmy Buffett
Copacabana (At the Copa) by Barry Manilow
Girls Just Want to Have Fun by Cyndi Lauper
I Go to Rio by Pablo Cruise
Istanbul (Not Constantinople) by Bart & Baker
Nobody by Sylvia
Oh Baby Mine (I Get so Lonely) by The Statler Brothers
Rhythm of the Night by DeBarge

10 Begin the Beguine by Richard Clayderman
Amame by Belle Perez
Have You Ever Seen the Rain by Creedence Clearwater Revival
(Sittin' on) the Dock of the Bay by Otis Redding
White Christmas by Kenny Vehkavaara

11 Blue Bayou by Linda Ronstadt
All I Have to Do Is Dream by The Everly Brothers
Grandpa (Tell Me 'Bout The Good Old Days) by The Judds
Grease by Frankie Valli
Green Green Grass of Home by Tom Jones
Gypsy Woman by Brian Hyland
Please Mr. Postman by The Marvelettes
Room Full of Roses by Mickey Gilley
Spanish Eyes by Bouke
The Ballad of the Green Berets by SSGT Barry Sadler
You Got It by Roy Orbison

12 Blueberry Hill by Fats Domino
After the Lovin' by Engelbert Humperdinck
Born Too Late by The Poni-Tails
Dream a Little Dream of Me by The Mamas & The Papas
Play That Song by Train
Summer Wind by Johnny Mercer
The Yellow Rose by Johnny Lee (with Lane Brody)
Till Then by The Mills Brothers

13 Boy from NYC by The Ad Libs
All I Want for Christmas is You by Vince Vance & The Valiants
Blame It on the Bossa Nova by Eydie Gorme
Coconut by Harry Nilsson
Everyday by Buddy Holly
Except for Monday by Lorrie Morgan
Feliz Navidad by Kenny Vehkavaara
Handy Man by Jimmy Jones
He's so Fine by The Chiffons
I Like It Like That by Chris Kenner
In the Summertime by Mungo Jerry
Let the Good Times Roll by Shirley & Lee
Little Darlin' by The Diamonds
Paint It, Black by The Rolling Stones
Papa Loves Mambo by Perry Como
Rockin' Around the Christmas Tree by Brenda Lee
Runaround Sue by Dion
Suspicion by Terry Stafford
Take Good Care of My Baby by Bobby Vee
Tweedle Dee by Georgia Gibbs
Twistin' the Night Away by Sam Cooke
Who Put the Bomp by Barry Mann
Will You Love Me Tomorrow by The Shirelles

14 Breaking Up Is Hard To Do by Neil Sedaka
Big Girls Don't Cry by Frankie Valli & The Four Seasons
Dream Lover by Bobby Darin
Johnny Angel by Shelley Fabares
Poison Ivy by The Coasters
Sherry by Frankie Valli & The Four Seasons
There Goes My Baby by The Drifters
Walk like a Man by Frankie Valli & The Four Seasons

15 Button Up Your Overcoat
by Miss Rose and Her Rhythm Percolators
Bye Bye Blackbird by The McGuire Sisters
Five Foot Two Eyes of Blue by Guy Lombardo
Honey Bun by Kelli O'Hara
It's Delovely by Anita O'Day
Meet Me Under the Mistletoe by Randy Travis
Pink Shoe Laces by Dodie Stevens
Plastic Jesus by Tia Blake

16 C'est Magnifique by Dean Martin
500 Miles Away from Home by Bobby Bare
A Love Worth Waiting for by Bouke
Pennies from Heaven by Paul Anka and Michael Buble

17 Cab Driver by The Mills Brothers
Buffalo Soldier by Bob Marley & The Wailers
Detroit City by Bobby Bare
Don't Fence Me In by Roy Rogers
Eighteen Wheels and A Dozen Roses by Kathy Mattea
Engine, Engine #9 by Roger Miller
'Lil Red Riding Hood by Sam The Sham & The Pharaohs
One Step Forward by The Desert Rose Band
Please Daddy (Don't Get Drunk This Christmas) by Alan Jackson
Rudolph the Red Nosed Reindeer by Burl Ives
'S Wonderful by The McGuire Sisters
Silver Bells by Lady Antebellum
Take These Chains from My Heart by Hank Williams
There's a Tear in My Beer
by Hank Williams Jr. (with Hank Williams)
Your Cheatin' Heart by Hank Williams and Drifting Cowboys

18 Chapel of Love by The Dixie Cups
Billie Jean by Michael Jackson
Green Onions by Booker T. & The M. G.'s
Mamma Maria by Ricchi E Poveri
Mary's Boy Child by Kensington Theatre Ensemble
My Guy by Mary Wells
Still the One by Orleans
The Letter by The Box Tops
Under the Boardwalk by The Drifters

19 Chihuahua by DJ Bobo
Bittersweet Samba by Herb Alpert & The Tijuana Brass
Dixie Road by Lee Greenwood
Escape (the Pina Colada Song) by Rupert Holmes
Every Little Step by Bobby Brown
Freddy My Love by Cindy Bullens
Hey Shango! by Squirrel Nut Zippers
I'm Yours by Jason Mraz
It's Only Make Believe by Tony Jackson
Limbo Rock by Herb Alpert & The Tijuana Brass
Little Bitty Pretty One by The Jackson 5
Mambo No. 5 by Lou Bega
Maneater by Daryl Hall & John Oates
Mariana Mambo by Chayanne
Penny Lover by Lionel Richie
Why Do Fools Fall in Love by Frankie Lymon & The Teenagers

20 Dance, Dance, Dance by The Beach Boys
Do You Love Me by The Contours

21 Dancing in the Street by Martha Reeves & The Vandellas
I Only Want You for Christmas by Alan Jackson
Signed, Sealed, Delivered (I'm Yours) by Stevie Wonder
The Best of My Love by The Emotions
Uptight (Everything's Alright) by Stevie Wonder
Where Did Our Love Go by The Supremes

22 Danke Schoen by Wayne Newton
Bring It On Home To Me by Sam Cooke
Don't Worry, Be Happy by Bobby McFarrin
Fishin' in the Dark by Nitty Gritty Dirt Band
Fooled Around and Fell in Love by Elvin Bishop
Hopelessly Devoted to You by Olivia Newton-John
Jamaica Farewell by Harry Belafonte
L-O-V-E by Nat King Cole
Mack the Knife by Bobby Darin
Sukiyaki by Kyu Sakamoto
Three Little Birds by Bob Marley & The Wailers
You Are My Sunshine by George Hamilton, IV

23 Do Ya' by K. T. Oslin
Billy Bayou by Roger Miller
Got No Reason Now For Goin' Home by Gene Watson
Help Me Make It Through the Night by Sammi Smith
You Make My Dreams Come True by The South Street Band

24 Don't Get Around Much Anymore by Anne Murray
Enjoy Yourself (It's Later Than You Think) by Guy Lombardo
Mame by Louis Armstrong

25 Don't It Make My Brown Eyes Blue by Crystal Gayle
Blue Christmas by Clay Walker
California Dreamin' by The Mamas & The Papas
Everything is Beautiful by Ray Stevens
Somethin' Stupid by Frank Sinatra and Nancy Sinatra
Winter Wonderland by Engelbert Humperdinck
You Are the Woman by Firefall
You Beat Me to the Punch by Mary Wells

26 Duke of Earl by Gene Chandler
Do You Remember Me by Santana
Hello My Name Is by Matthew West
I Want a Hippopotamus for Christmas by Gayla Peevey
Missing You by John Waite
One of These Nights by The Eagles
Rock with You by Michael Jackson

27 Everybody's Somebody's Fool by Connie Francis
Afternoon Delight by Starland Vocal Band
Bitty Boppy Betty by Pink Martini
Bread & Butter by The Newbeats
Cheek to Cheek by Fred Astaire
Cotton Fields by Creedence Clearwater Revival
Exes and Ohs by The Nicol Kings
Move It on Over by Hank Williams
Palisades Park by Freddy Cannon
Roll Back The Rug by Scooter Lee
Sweet Soul Music by Arthur Conley

28 Family Tradition by Hank Williams, Jr.
Achy Breaky Heart by Billy Ray Cyrus
An American Dream by Nitty Gritty Dirt Band
Between Winston-Salem and Nashville Tennessee
by The Mills Brothers
Elvira by The Oak Ridge Boys
Grapefruit – Juicy Fruit by Jimmy Buffett
I Can Help by Billy Swan
I Got Mexico by Eddy Raven
Just Call Me Lonesome by Radney Foster
Love Drunk by LOCASH
Margaritaville by Jimmy Buffett
My Maria by Brooks & Dunn
Pick Me Up on Your Way Down by The Tractors
Rock Me Gently by Andy Kim
Show Me the Way by Peter Frampton
Woman by Mark Chesnutt

29 Fascination by Al Martino
Believe Me If All Those Endearing Young Charms
by Brian Coll
He'll Have to Go by Jim Reeves
I Wonder Who's Kissing Her Now by Harry Nilsson
Les Bicyclettes de Belsize by Engelbert Humperdinck
Silent Night by REO Speedwagon
The Last Waltz by Engelbert Humperdinck
Unchained Melody by Gold Star Ballroom Orchestra

30 Forever and Ever Amen by Randy Travis
Blue Christmas by John Anderson
Everybody by DJ BoBo and INNA
I've Got a Tiger by the Tail by Buck Owens
It Must be Love by Don Williams
Just My Imagination (Running Away with Me)
by The Temptations
Land of Enchantment by Michael Martin Murphey
Love Letters in the Sand by Pat Boone
On the Other Hand by Randy Travis
Straight to Hell by Drivin N Cryin

31 Gentle on My Mind by The Band Perry
All I Have to Do Is Dream by Anne Murray
Every Time You Go Away by Paul Young
Gypsy Queen by Chris Norman
How Great Thou Art by Alan Jackson
I Was Country When Country Wasn't Cool
by Barbara Mandrell and George Jones
I Wonder Who's Kissing Her Now by Dean Martin
If You Don't Wanna See Santa Claus Cry by Alan Jackson
Reminiscing by Little River Band
Silent Night by Kenny Vehkavaara
Silver Bells by Kenny Vehkavaara
Some Enchanted Evening by The Temptations
The Christmas Song by Kenny Vehkavaara
The Riddle Song by Sam Cooke
Veneno by Danny Ocean
White Christmas by Elvis Presley

32 Glow Worm by The Mills Brothers
C'est La Vie by Emmylou Harris
Forget Him by Bobby Rydell
Island Song by Zac Brown Band
One Love/People Get Ready by Bob Marley & The Wailers
One Toke over the Line by Brewer & Shipley
There's a Kind of Hush by The Carpenters

33 Goody, Goody by Ella Fitzgerald
Every Breath You Take by The Police
From a Jack to a King by Ricky Van Shelton
Good Directions by Billy Currington
It's a Good Day by Peggy Lee
Montego Bay by Bobby Bloom
Pretty Blue Eyes by Steve Lawrence and Eydie Gorme
Shambala by Three Dog Night
Stand by Me by Ben E. King

34 Harper Valley PTA by Jeannie C. Riley
39-21-46 by General Johnson & The Chairmen of the Board
Adouma by Santana
Almost Jamaica by The Bellamy Brothers
Candida by Tony Orlando and Dawn
Come Dance with Me by Nancy Hays
I Love a Rainy Night by Eddie Rabbitt
It's Now or Never by Elvis Presley
Kokomo by The Beach Boys
Let It Snow by Papi Gonzalez
My Boyfriend's Back by The Angels
Rockin' Around the Christmas Tree by Jack Jezzro
Spanish Harlem by Ben E. King
Summer Nights by John Travolta and Olivia Newton-John
That'll Be the Day by Buddy Holly & The Crickets

35 Heaven's Just a Sin Away by The Kendalls
Get Your Kicks on Route 66 by Asleep at the Wheel
Java by Al Hirt
One Fine Day by The Chiffons
Ooh La La by Faces
So into You by Atlanta Rhythm Section
Walk of Life by Dire Straits

36 I Believe in You by Don Williams
Across the Bridge by Jim Reeves
Dance Above the Rainbow by Ronan Hardiman
Deep in the Heart of Texas by American Patriots
Don't Close Your Eyes by Keith Whitley
Good Hearted Woman by Waylon Jennings
Grandma Got Run Over by a Reindeer by Elmo & Patsy
Hello Walls by Faron Young
Hey, Soul Sister by Train
Highway 40 Blues by Ricky Skaggs
If You've Got the Money by Lefty Frizzell
In the Shade of the Old Apple Tree
by Louis Armstrong and The Mills Brothers
Just to See You Smile by Tim McGraw
Six Days on the Road by Dave Dudley
Swing Baby by David Ball
The Chair by George Strait
The Yellow Rose of Texas by Roy Rogers
(There's) No Getting' Over Me by Ronnie Milsap
Too Old to Cut the Mustard by Red Foley and Ernest Tubb
Top of the World by The Carpenters
Who's in the Strawberry Patch with Sally
by Tony Orlando and Dawn

37 I Can't Help Myself (Sugar Pie, Honey Bunch) by Four Tops
Get Down Tonight by KC & The Sunshine Band
It Don't Come Easy by Ringo Starr
Rag Doll by Frankie Valli
This Old Heart of Mine (Is Weak for You) by The Isley Brothers
Wouldn't It Be Nice by The Beach Boys

38 I Do, I Do, I Do, I Do by ABBA
I Can't Help It If I'm Still in Love with You by Linda Ronstadt
Walk Away Renee by Four Tops

39 (I Don't Know Why) But I Do by Clarence "Frogman" Henry
A Fool Such as I by Willie Nelson and Hank Snow
Dream a Little Dream by Robbie Williams and Lily Allen
Whiskey Bent and Hell Bound by Hank Williams, Jr.

40 I'm Looking over a Four Leaf Clover by Mitch Miller
Everybody Loves My Baby by Bing Crosby
Pay Me Now (or Pay Me Later) by Squirrel Nut Zippers
Put a Lid on It by Squirrel Nut Zippers
Salty Dog Rag by Eddie Hill
The Vatican Rag by Stargazers

41 I'm so Lonesome I Could Cry by Hank Williams
Here's a Quarter (Call Someone Who Cares) by Travis Tritt
Home on the Range by Gene Autry
The Rock and Roll Waltz by Kay Starr
Waltz Across Texas by Ernest Tubb
You Look so Good in Love by George Strait

42 In Search of Mona Lisa by Santana
Butterflies by Michael Jackson
Drink in My Hand by Eric Church
Game of Love by Santana (with Tina Turner)
Hot Stuff by Donna Summer
Last Christmas by Wham!
Listen to the Rhythm of the Falling Rain by Johnny Tillotson
Lonely Town by Theo Katzman and Vulfpeck
My Prerogative by Bobby Brown
Swing Low Sweet Chariot by Johnny Cash
The Way You Make Me Feel by Michael Jackson

43 In the Garden by Alan Jackson
Amazing Grace by Reba McEntire
Could I Have This Dance by Frankie McBride
It's a Sin to Tell a Lie by Ann Breen
Let There Be Peace on Earth by Bill & Gloria Gaither
Try to Remember by Patti Page

44 In the Mood by Glenn Miller
Bei Mir Bist Du Schon by Girls From Mars
I'm so Excited by The Pointer Sisters
Louisiana Saturday Night by Mel McDaniel

45 Inishannon Serenade by Frank Chacksfield
Blue Night by Michael Learns To Rock
It's Too Late by Carole King
Me and My Shadow by Julie London
Nothing's Gonna Stop Us Now by Starship
Perhaps, Perhaps, Perhaps by Doris Day
Stand by Your Man by Tammy Wynette
Take My Breath Away by Berlin
Who's Sorry Now by Connie Francis

46 Islands in the Stream by Dolly Parton and Kenny Rogers
Last Christmas by Glee Cast
Louie, Louie by The Kingsmen
Love Grows (Where My Rosemary Goes) by Edison Lighthouse
To Love Somebody by The Bee Gees
You're the One That I Want
by John Travolta and Olivia Newton-John

47 It Had to Be You by John Stevens
Another Saturday Night by Sam Cooke
I'm Too Sexy for My Shirt by Gliese
King of the Road by Roger Miller
Pink Panther Theme by Henry Mancini
Theme from New York, New York by Frank Sinatra
We Need a Little Christmas by Johnny Mathis

48 Karma Chameleon by Culture Club
Ain't No Woman (Like the One I've Got) by Four Tops
Beauty School Dropout by Frankie Avalon
Bette Davis Eyes by Kim Carnes
Blame It on the Boogie by The Jacksons
Do That to Me One More Time by Captain & Tennille
Flowers on the Wall by The Statler Brothers
I'm Stone in Love with You by The Stylistics
Jingle Bells by Kenny Vehkavaara
Listen to the Music by The Doobie Brothers
On the Road Again by Willie Nelson
Rhinestone Cowboy by Glen Campbell
What's Love Got to Do with It by Tina Turner
Winter Wonderland by Kenny Vehkavaara

49 Love Train by The O Jays
Baby I Need Your Loving by Four Tops
Beer Barrel Polka by Bobby Vinton
Give Me Just a Little More Time
by General Johnson & The Chairmen of the Board
Lovesick Blues by Hank Williams
Michael Row the Boat Ashore by The Highway Men
Mother-In-Law by Ernie K-Doe
Pennsylvania Polka by Bobby Vinton
Please Help Me, I'm Falling by Hank Locklin
Sooner or Later by The Grass Roots
Sugar, Sugar by The Archies

50 Mambo Italiano by Bette Midler
Bobby's Girl by Marcie Blane
Frosty the Snowman by Kenny Vehkavaara
Lollipop by the Chordettes
People Will Say We're in Love
by Bing Crosby and Rosemary Clooney
Rockin' with the Rhythm of the Rain by The Judds
Save the Last Dance for Me by The Drifters
Welcome to Burlesque by Cher
Who Did You Call Darlin' by Heather Myles

51 Midnight Train to Georgia by Gladys Knight & The Pips
A Horse with No Name by America
Let's Stay Together by Al Green
Southern Nights by Glen Campbell
What Becomes of the Brokenhearted by Jimmy Ruffin

52 Mockingbird by Carly Simon and James Taylor
A Place in the Sun by Stevie Wonder
Abilene by George Hamilton IV
Baby It's Cold Outside by Margaret Whiting and Johnny Mercer
Blood is Thicker than Water by Eddie Floyd
Calendar Girl by Neil Sedaka
I Saw Mommy Kissing Santa Claus by The Jackson 5
Meat and Potato Man by Alan Jackson

53 Molly Malone by The Dubliners
Are You Lonesome Tonight by Anne Murray
Don't We All Have the Right by Ricky Van Shelton
I Forgot More Than You'll Ever Know by Skeeter Davis
I Wonder Who's Kissing Him Now by Anne Murray
If My Heart Had Windows by Patty Loveless
Pretty Paper by Randy Travis
Take My Hand, Precious Lord by Jim Reeves

54 Mr. Sandman by The Chordettes
Build Me Up Buttercup by The Foundations
Diana by Paul Anka
Jingle Bell Rock by Jack Jezzro and Sam Levine
Joy to the World by Three Dog Night
Kansas City by Wilbert Harrison
Oh Carol by Neil Sedaka
Poetry in Motion by Johnny Tillotson
School Day by Chuck Berry
That's Why (I Love You So) by Jackie Wilson

55 My Girl by The Temptations
Don't Worry Baby by The Beach Boys
How Sweet It Is (To Be Loved By You) by Marvin Gaye
Nevertheless (I'm in Love with You) by The Mills Brothers
Pretty Little Angel Eyes by Curtiss Lee
Sleigh Ride by Kenny Vehkavaara
Stop! In the Name of Love by The Supremes
Sunshine of Your Love by Cream

56 No No Song by Ringo Starr
Happy Together by The Turtles
My Blue Heaven by John Stevens
Sh Boom (Life Could Be a Dream) by The Crew Cuts
Spirit in the Sky by Norman Greenbaum
Tiny Bubbles by The Mills Brothers
Tip Toe Through the Tulips by The McGuire Sisters
Uptown Funk by Mark Ransom and Bruno Mars

57 Poor Little Fool by Ricky Nelson
I Second That Emotion by Smokey Robinson & The Miracles
Mele Kalikimaka by Jimmy Buffett
Only You (And You Alone) by The Platters
Standing in the Shadows of Love by Four Tops
Steamroller Blues by Elvis Presley
Sweet Home Alabama by Lynyrd Skynyrd
Understand Your Man by Johnny Cash

58 Ready to Roll by Blake Shelton
Bye, Bye Love by The Everly Brothers
Dominique by The Singing Nuns
He Ain't Heavy He's My Brother by The Hollies
Hungry Eyes by Eric Carmen
It's Gonna Rain by Charles Johnson
Make Love to Me by Anne Murray
Midnight Blue by Melissa Manchester
Santa Bring My Baby Back to Me by Elvis Presley
Santa Claus is Coming to Town by Dolly Parton
Volcano by Jimmy Buffett
Wake Up Little Susie by The Everly Brothers
What Christmas Means to Me by Jessica Simpson
You Make It Feel like Christmas
by Gwen Stefani and Blake Shelton

59 Release Me by The Mills Brothers
Ain't Misbehavin', by Hank Williams, Jr.
Do You Remember These? by The Statler Brothers
Only You (And You Alone) by Ringo Starr
You Sexy Thing by Hot Chocolate
You've Got a Friend by James Taylor
You've Got a Friend in Me by Lyle Lovett and Randy Newman

60 Seven Year Ache by Rosanne Cash
Brandy by Looking Glass
It's a Heartache by Bonnie Tyler
Sandy by John Travolta
Some Beach by Blake Shelton
(Up A) Lazy River by The Mills Brothers

61 Silhouettes by The Rays
God Rest Ye Merry Gentlemen by Kenny Vehkavaara
I Think I Love You by The Partridge Family
Stayin' Alive by Bee Gees
The Great Pretender by The Platters
Twilight Time by The Platters
You Made Me Love You by Patsy Cline

62 Sixteen Candles by The Crests
Baby Come Back by Player
Because by The Dave Clark Five
It's Only Make Believe by Conway Twitty
Love is Here and Now You're Gone by The Supremes
Merry Christmas Everyone by Shakin Stevens
Proud Mary by Creedence Clearwater Revival
The Tracks of My Tears by Smokey Robinson & The Miracles

63 Soldier Boy by The Shirelles
Dance with Me by Orleans
I Just Want to Dance with You by George Strait
I'm a Fool to Care by Boz Scaggs
Is This Love by Bob Marley & The Wailers
Jimmy Mack by Martha Reeves and The Vandellas
Just One Look by Linda Ronstadt
Pretty Belinda by Chris Andrews
So Sad (To Watch Good Love Go Bad) by The Everly Brothers
We'll Sing in the Sunshine by Gale Garnett
Winter Wonderland by Brad Paisley

64 Something's Gotta Give by The McGuire Sisters
A Little Bit Independent by Gene Merlino, Diana Lee,
and Shep Fields & His Rippling Rhythm
Ain't She Sweet by Frank Sinatra
Fugue for Tinhorns by Barry Manilow
Hey Good Lookin' by Hank Williams
I Fall to Pieces by Patsy Cline
I've Got My Love to Keep Me Warm by The Mills Brothers
I've Got You Under My Skin by Frank Sinatra
Maggie May by Rod Stewart
Sweet Little Liza by Major Dundee Band with Dick Van Altena
The Girl from Ipanema by Steve Lawrence and Eydie Gorme
The Way You Look Tonight by Frank Sinatra
Yes Sir! That's My Baby by Bing Crosby

65 Soul Man by Sam & Dave
A Hundred Pounds of Clay by Gene McDaniels
It's All Right by The Impressions
Just One Look by Doris Troy
Lucille by The Everly Brothers
Poor Side of Town by Del Shannon
Poor Side of Town by Johnny Rivers
Spooky by Classics IV

66 Swingin' by John Anderson
Girl Watcher by The New Summer Fun Project
Happy Trails by Roy Rogers and Dale Evans
If You Change Your Mind by Roseanne Cash
Jambalaya (On The Bayou) by Nitty Gritty Dirt Band
Jingle Bell Rock by Bobby Helms
Milk Cow Blues by George Strait
Put Another Log on the Fire by The Geezinslaws
Rambling Rose by Floyd Burton
Right or Wrong by George Strait
Streets of Bakersfield by Buck Owens
This Guy's in Love with You by Herb Alpert & The Tijuana Brass
This Little Light of Mine by Sam Cooke
Tulsa Time by Don Williams

67 Take a Chance on Me by ABBA
Beast of Burden by The Rolling Stones
Hit the Road, Jack by Omar and The Howlers
I Will Follow Him by Little Peggy Marsh
Mary's Boy Child by Boney M.
Put a Little Love in Your Heart by Jackie DeShannon
When You're in Love with a Beautiful Woman by Dr. Hook
You're so Vain by Carly Simon

68 Tennessee Waltz by Patti Page
Hello Darlin' by Conway Twitty
Rose Colored Glasses by John Conlee
There Goes My Everything by Anne Murray

69 Tequila by The Champs
Runaway by Del Shannon
Sweet Nothin's by Brenda Lee

70 The Lion Sleeps Tonight (Wimoweh) by The Tokens
Needles and Pins by The Searchers
Walk Right Back by The Everly Brothers
Working My Way Back to You by The Spinners

71 The Wanderer by Dion
A Holly Jolly Christmas by Alan Jackson
Bad Bad Leroy Brown by Jim Croce
It's My Party by Lesley Gore
Let's Hang On by Frankie Valli
Mustang Sally by Wilson Pickett
Stagger Lee by Lloyd Price
The Blues Is Alright by Little Milton
When Will I See You Again by Three Degrees

72 Uptown by Roy Orbison
Come Go with Me by The Del-Vikings
Everybody's Talkin' by Harry Nilsson

73 Western Girls by Marty Stuart
Burning Love by Elvis Presley
Honky Tonk Christmas by Alan Jackson
Shop Around by The Miracles

74 Y'all Come Back Saloon by The Oak Ridge Boys
I'm Just an Old Chunk of Coal by John Anderson
One Night at a Time by George Strait
This Little Light of Mine by Brenda Lee with Charlie Daniels

75 You're Nobody 'til Somebody Loves You by Dean Martin
Heart and Soul by Al Alberts and The Four Aces
I'm Gonna Sit Right Down and Write Myself a Letter
by Sir Paul McCartney
It Never Rains in Southern California by Albert Hammond
Rhythm of the Rain by The Cascades
Rose Garden by Lynn Anderson
You Make Me Feel so Young by Frank Sinatra

THEMED PLAYLISTS

A FOOL'S PARADISE
54 **Build Me Up Buttercup** by The Foundations
54 **Oh Carol** by Neil Sedaka
4 **Cathy's Clown** by The Everly Brothers
61 **The Great Pretender** by The Platters
61 **You Made Me Love You** by Patsy Cline
71 **It's My Party** by Lesley Gore
62 **It's Only Make Believe** by Conway Twitty
57 **Poor Little Fool** by Ricky Nelson
57 **Standing in the Shadows of Love** by Four Tops
30 **Love Letters in the Sand** by Pat Boone

A LITTLE OF THIS
52 **Mockingbird** by Carly Simon and James Taylor
56 **Tip Toe Through the Tulips** by The McGuire Sisters
15 **Plastic Jesus** by Tia Blake
50 **Mambo Italiano** by Bette Midler
13 **Blame It on the Bossa Nova** by Eydie Gorme
1 **Neon Moon** by Brooks & Dunn
23 **Billy Bayou** by Roger Miller
33 **Stand by Me** by Ben E. King

A LITTLE OF THAT
42 **My Prerogative** by Bobby Brown
40 **Salty Dog Rag** by Eddie Hill
64 **A Little Bit Independent** by Gene Merlino, Diana Lee,
and Shep Fields & His Rippling Rhythm
47 **Theme from New York, New York** by Frank Sinatra
49 **Love Train by The O Jays**
12 **Play That Song** by Train
9 **Alley Cat** by Chet Atkins
19 **Chihuahua** by DJ BoBo

AS TIME GOES BY
40 **I'm Looking over a Four Leaf Clover** by Mitch Miller
59 **You Sexy Thing** by Hot Chocolate
5 **All of Me** by Michael Buble
51 **Let's Stay Together** by Al Green
22 **Danke Schoen** by Wayne Newton
46 **Islands in the Stream** by Dolly Parton and Kenny Rogers
35 **Ooh La La** by Faces
43 **Try to Remember** by Patti Page

ATTITUDE OF GRATITUDE
66 **This Little Light of Mine** by Sam Cooke
13 **Everyday** by Buddy Holly
22 **Sukiyaki** by Kyu Sakamoto
15 **It's Delovely** by Anita O'Day
3 **On the Sunny Side of the Street**
by Tony Bennett and Willie Nelson
59 **Do You Remember These?** by The Statler Brothers
56 **Uptown Funk** by Mark Ronson and Bruno Mars
29 **Fascination** by Al Martino

BURN THE FLOOR
20 **Dance, Dance, Dance** by The Beach Boys
21 **Dancing in the Street** by Martha Reeves & The Vandellas
37 **Get Down Tonight** by KC & The Sunshine Band
71 **Mustang Sally** by Wilson Pickett
61 **Stayin' Alive** by Bee Gees
57 **Steamroller Blues** by Elvis Presley
46 **You're the One That I Want**
by John Travolta and Olivia Newton-John
27 **Roll Back the Rug** by Scooter Lee
13 **Who Put the Bomp** by Barry Mann

COLOR ME
36 **The Yellow Rose of Texas** by Roy Rogers
15 **Bye Bye Blackbird** by The McGuire Sisters
25 **Don't It Make My Brown Eyes Blue** by Crystal Gayle
12 **Blueberry Hill** by Fats Domino
45 **Blue Night** by Michael Learns To Rock
48 **Karma Chameleon** by Culture Club
7 **Red Roses for a Blue Lady** by Johnny Tillotson
66 **Rambling Rose** by Floyd Burton
68 **Rose Colored Glasses** by John Conlee

COUNTRY AS CAN BE
34 **I Love a Rainy Night** by Eddie Rabbitt
22 **Fishin' in the Dark** by Nitty Gritty Dirt Band
66 **Swingin'** by John Anderson
6 **Trashy Women** by Confederate Railroad
74 **Y'all Come Back Saloon** by The Oak Ridge Boys
60 **It's a Heartache** by Bonnie Tyler
45 **Stand by Your Man** by Tammy Wynette
41 **Waltz Across Texas** by Ernest Tubb

DREAMIN'
1 **Over the Rainbow** by Israel Ka'ano'i Kamakawiwo'ole
39 **Dream a Little Dream** by Robbie Williams and Lily Allen
31 **All I Have to Do Is Dream** by Anne Murray
28 **An American Dream** by Nitty Gritty Dirt Band
34 **Almost Jamaica** by The Bellamy Brothers
25 **California Dreamin'** by The Mamas & The Papas
60 **(Up A) Lazy River** by The Mills Brothers
50 **Welcome to Burlesque** by Cher
23 **You Make My Dreams Come True** by The South Street Band
52 **A Place in the Sun** by Stevie Wonder

FACTS OF LIFE
6 **Viva La Vida** by Coldplay
34 **Harper Valley P.T.A.** by Jeannie C. Riley
47 **Another Saturday Night** by Sam Cooke
28 **Family Tradition** by Hank Williams, Jr.
22 **Don't Worry, Be Happy** by Bobby McFarrin
24 **Enjoy Yourself (It's Later Than You Think)** by Guy Lombardo
2 **The Same Way You Came In** by Big Tom
17 **Eighteen Wheels and A Dozen Roses** by Kathy Mattea
53 **Molly Malone** by The Dubliners

GAME OF LOVE
45 **Perhaps, Perhaps, Perhaps** by Doris Day
39 **(I Don't Know Why) But I Do** by Clarence "Frogman" Henry
59 **Ain't Misbehavin'** by Hank Williams, Jr.
18 **Chapel of Love** by The Dixie Cups
35 **Heaven's Just a Sin Away** by The Kendalls
30 **On the Other Hand** by Randy Travis
66 **Put Another Log on the Fire** by The Geezinslaws
27 **Move It on Over** by Hank Williams
17 **There's a Tear in My Beer** by Hank Williams, Jr.
23 **Do Ya'** by K. T. Oslin

GETTING' BETTER ALL THE TIME
74 **I'm Just an Old Chunk of Coal** by John Anderson
2 **Act Naturally** by Buck Owens
3 **Ain't That a Kick in the Head** by Dean Martin
17 **'S Wonderful** by The McGuire Sisters
26 **One of These Nights** by The Eagles
7 **I'll Get Over You** by Helen McCaffrey
45 **Nothing's Gonna Stop Us Now** by Starship
59 **You've Got a Friend** by James Taylor

GOIN' PLACES
34 **Candida** by Tony Orlando and Dawn
72 **Uptown** by Roy Orbison
47 **King of the Road** by Roger Miller
35 **Get Your Kicks on Route 66** by Asleep at the Wheel
17 **Don't Fence Me In** by Roy Rogers
28 **Margaritaville** by Jimmy Buffett
32 **One Toke over the Line** by Brewer & Shipley
51 **Midnight Train to Georgia** by Gladys Knight & The Pips
58 **Volcano** by Jimmy Buffett

IN A LONE STAR STATE OF MIND
6 **All My Exes Live in Texas** by George Strait
52 **Abilene** by George Hamilton IV
36 **Deep in the Heart of Texas** by American Patriots
36 **The Yellow Rose of Texas** by Roy Rogers
12 **The Yellow Rose** by Johnny Lee (with Lane Brody)
48 **Rhinestone Cowboy** by Glen Campbell
41 **Home on the Range** by Gene Autry
41 **Waltz Across Texas** by Ernest Tubb

LAW OF ATTRACTION
8 **Big Spender** by Peggy Lee
13 **Boy from NYC** by The Ad Libs
24 **Mame** by Louis Armstrong
63 **Just One Look** by Linda Ronstadt
46 **You're the One That I Want** by John Travolta and
Olivia Newton-John
36 **Hey, Soul Sister** by Train
19 **Mariana Mambo** by Chayanne
39 **(I Don't Know Why) But I Do** by Clarence "Frogman" Henry
29 **The Last Waltz** by Engelbert Humperdinck

LET'S BIG APPLE
13 **Boy from NYC** by The Ad Libs
65 **Poor Side of Town** by Del Shannon
34 **Spanish Harlem** by Ben E. King
47 **Theme from New York, New York** by Frank Sinatra
72 **Uptown** by Roy Orbison
56 **Uptown Funk** by Mark Ronson and Bruno Mars
7 **Anything Goes** by Frank Sinatra
36 **If You've Got The Money** by Lefty Frizzell

LOST AND FOUND
36 **Hello Walls** by Faron Young
28 **Show Me The Way** by Peter Frampton
40 **I'm Looking over a Four Leaf Clover** by Mitch Miller
66 **If You Change Your Mind** by Roseanne Cash
56 **Spirit in the Sky** by Norman Greenbaum
74 **This Little Light of Mine** by Brenda Lee with Charlie Daniels
26 **Hello My Name Is** by Matthew West
31 **How Great Thou Art** by Alan Jackson

LOVE GONE
12 **Summer Wind** by Johnny Mercer
39 **A Fool Such as I** by Willie Nelson and Hank Snow
17 **Engine, Engine #9** by Roger Miller
33 **Goody, Goody** by Ella Fitzgerald
45 **Who's Sorry Now** by Connie Francis
24 **Don't Get Around Much Anymore** by Anne Murray
6 **All My Exes Live in Texas** by George Strait
2 **Oh Lonesome Me** by Don Gibson
53 **I Forgot More Than You'll Ever Know** by Skeeter Davis

LOVE POTION
13 **Blame It on the Bossa Nova** by Eydie Gorme
56 **Tiny Bubbles** by The Mills Brothers
32 **There's a Kind of Hush** by The Carpenters
5 **Fly Me to the Moon** by Scooter Lee
48 **I'm Stone in Love with You** by The Stylistics
1 **Amor** by Eydie Gorme and Los Panchos
22 **L-O-V-E** by Nat King Cole
16 **C'est Magnifique** by Dean Martin
50 **Lollipop** by The Chordettes

LOVE UNREQUITED
12 **Born Too Late** by The Poni-Tails
19 **It's Only Make Believe** by Tony Jackson
7 **On the Street Where You Live** by Dean Martin
35 **So into You** by Atlanta Rhythm Section
27 **Everybody's Somebody's Fool** by Connie Francis
9 **Oh Baby Mine (I Get so Lonely)** by The Statler Brothers
60 **Seven Year Ache** by Rosanne Cash
41 **I'm so Lonesome I Could Cry** by Hank Williams

LOVEY DOVEY
1 A Kiss to Build a Dream on by Louis Armstrong
63 I Just Want to Dance with You by George Strait
5 All I Do Is Dream of You by Michael Bublé
75 You Make Me Feel so Young by Frank Sinatra
12 Play That Song by Train
47 It Had to Be You by John Stevens
59 Only You (And You Alone) by Ringo Starr
36 I Believe in You by Don Williams
41 You Look so Good in Love by George Strait

(MIS)BEHAVIN'
19 Mambo No. 5 by Lou Bega
28 Grapefruit – Juicy Fruit by Jimmy Buffett
30 Straight to Hell by Drivin N Cryin
42 Drink in My Hand by Eric Church
39 Whiskey Bent and Hell Bound by Hank Williams, Jr.
40 Put a Lid on It by Squirrel Nut Zippers
60 Seven Year Ache by Rosanne Cash
22 Fooled Around and Fell in Love by Elvin Bishop
36 Who's in the Strawberry Patch with Sally
by Tony Orlando and Dawn

MISSIN' MY BABY
11 Blue Bayou by Linda Ronstadt
59 Release Me by The Mills Brothers
17 Take These Chains from My Heart by Hank Williams
8 I Can't Help It If I'm Still in Love with You by Linda Ronstadt
42 Listen to the Rhythm of the Falling Rain by Johnny Tillotson
22 Bring It On Home To Me by Sam Cooke
13 Except for Monday by Lorrie Morgan
28 I Got Mexico by Eddy Raven
68 Tennessee Waltz by Patti Page

ON CLOUD NINE
11 You Got It by Roy Orbison
18 Chapel of Love by The Dixie Cups
57 I Second That Emotion by Smokey Robinson & The Miracles
15 It's Delovely by Anita O'Day
54 Joy to the World by Three Dog Night
7 Let Your Love Flow by The Bellamy Brothers
58 Ready to Roll by Blake Shelton
36 Top of the World by The Carpenters

PEDAL THE METAL
25 **California Dreamin'** by The Mamas & The Papas
28 **Between Winston-Salem and Nashville Tennessee**
by The Mills Brothers
35 **Get Your Kicks on Route 66** by Asleep at the Wheel
30 **Land of Enchantment** by Michael Martin Murphey
44 **Louisiana Saturday Night** by Mel McDaniel
36 **Six Days on the Road** by Dave Dudley
66 **Tulsa Time** by Don Williams
17 **Eighteen Wheels and A Dozen Roses** by Kathy Mattea

PURE JOY
27 **Afternoon Delight** by Starland Vocal Band
10 **Begin the Beguine** by Richard Clayderman
52 **Calendar Girl** by Neil Sedaka
18 **My Guy** by Mary Wells
63 **Soldier Boy** by The Shirelles
34 **Summer Nights** by John Travolta and Olivia Newton-John
25 **You Beat Me to the Punch** by Mary Wells
22 **You Are My Sunshine** by George Hamilton, IV
55 **Sunshine of Your Love** by Cream

READY FOR LOVE
3 **Singin' in the Rain** by Doris Day
10 **Begin the Beguine** by Richard Clayderman
44 **In the Mood** by Glenn Miller
64 **Hey Good Lookin'** by Hank Williams
67 **Take a Chance on Me** by ABBA
27 **Afternoon Delight** by Starland Vocal Band
34 **It's Now or Never** by Elvis Presley
31 **Gentle on My Mind** by The Band Perry

RIBBONS OF HIGHWAY
71 **The Wanderer** by Dion
19 **Dixie Road** by Lee Greenwood
67 **Hit the Road, Jack** by Omar and The Howlers
47 **King of the Road** by Roger Miller
54 **Kansas City** by Wilbert Harrison
42 **Lonely Town** by Theo Katzman and Vulfpeck
32 **One Toke over the Line** by Brewer & Shipley
48 **On the Road Again** by Willie Nelson
57 **Sweet Home Alabama** by Lynyrd Skynyrd

STARFISH & PINEAPPLE
32 **Island Song** by Zac Brown Band
46 **Islands in the Stream** by Dolly Parton and Kenny Rogers
34 **Kokomo** by The Beach Boys
3 **Red Sails in the Sunset** by Johnny Lee
60 **Sandy** by John Travolta
10 **(Sittin' on) the Dock of the Bay** by Otis Redding
22 **Jamaica Farewell** by Harry Belafonte
71 **When Will I See You Again** by Three Degrees
59 **You Sexy Thing** by Hot Chocolate

STRUTTIN' THE STUFF
32 **Glow Worm** by The Mills Brothers
66 **This Little Light of Mine** by Sam Cooke
64 **Ain't She Sweet** by Frank Sinatra
8 **A White Sport Coat (and A Pink Carnation)** by Marty Robbins
15 **Pink Shoe Laces** by Dodie Stevens
47 **I'm Too Sexy for My Shirt** by Gliese
67 **You're so Vain** by Carly Simon
36 **If You've Got the Money** by Lefty Frizzell
40 **The Vatican Rag** by Stargazers

SWEET SOMETHINGS
15 **Honey Bun** by Kelli O'Hara
55 **How Sweet It Is (To Be Loved By You)** by Marvin Gaye
50 **Lollipop** by The Chordettes
14 **Sherry** by Frankie Valli & The Four Seasons
49 **Sugar, Sugar** by The Archies
3 **Sugar Shack** by Jimmy Gilmer & The Fireballs
64 **Sweet Little Liza** by Major Dundee Band with Dick Van Altena
27 **Sweet Soul Music** by Arthur Conley

TAKE ME HOME
36 **The Chair** by George Strait
7 **On the Street Where You Live** by Dean Martin
1 **Walkin' My Baby Back Home** by Nat King Cole
56 **My Blue Heaven** by John Stevens
23 **Got No Reason Now For Goin' Home** by Gene Watson
5 **Show Me the Way to Go Home** by Jimmy and the Parrots
42 **Swing Low Sweet Chariot** by Johnny Cash
11 **Green Green Grass of Home** by Tom Jones
41 **Home on the Range** by Gene Autry
75 **It Never Rains in Southern California** by Albert Hammond

TOES IN THE WATER
42 Drink in My Hand by Eric Church
64 The Girl from Ipanema by Steve Lawrence and Eydie Gorme
66 Girl Watcher by The New Summer Fun Project
54 Poetry in Motion by Johnny Tillotson
56 Sh Boom (Life Could Be a Dream) by The Crew Cuts
28 Margaritaville by Jimmy Buffett
1 Neon Moon by Brooks & Dunn
33 Montego Bay by Bobby Bloom
60 Some Beach by Blake Shelton

TRUE LOVE
75 You're Nobody 'til Somebody Loves You by Dean Martin
44 Bei Mir Bist Du Schon by Girls From Mars
38 I Do, I Do, I Do, I Do by ABBA
32 C'est La Vie by Emmylou Harris
46 Love Grows (Where My Rosemary Goes)
by Edison Lighthouse
30 Forever and Ever Amen by Randy Travis
1 True Love Ways by Mickey Gilley
43 Could I Have This Dance by Frankie McBride

WATCH OUT
22 Mack the Knife by Bobby Darin
2 Bad Moon Rising by Creedence Clearwater Revival
31 Gypsy Queen by Chris Norman
9 Nobody by Sylvia
56 No No Song by Ringo Starr
49 Mother-In-Law by Ernie K-Doe
27 Move It on Over by Hank Williams
17 Your Cheatin' Heart by Hank Williams and Drifting Cowboys
68 Tennessee Waltz by Patti Page

WOK TALK & LIQUID EDIBLES
27 Bread & Butter by The Newbeats
60 Brandy by Looking Glass
13 Coconut by Harry Nilsson
11 Grease by Frankie Valli
18 Green Onions by Booker T. & The M. G.'s
28 Grapefruit – Juicy Fruit by Jimmy Buffett
66 Jambalaya (On The Bayou) by Nitty Gritty Dirt Band
35 Java by Al Hirt
69 Tequila by The Champs

WORKIN' IT
64 **Fugue for Tinhorns** by Barry Manilow
17 **Buffalo Soldier** by Bob Marley & The Wailers
42 **Lonely Town** by Theo Katzman and Vulfpeck
6 **Working in the Coal Mine** by Lee Dorsey
27 **Cotton Fields** by Creedence Clearwater Revival
40 **Pay Me Now (or Pay Me Later)** by Squirrel Nut Zippers
58 **Ready to Roll** by Blake Shelton
36 **Swing Baby** by David Ball

FOR CHRISTMAS:

SANTA BABY
52 **Baby It's Cold Outside** by Margaret Whiting and
Johnny Mercer
1 **Santa Baby** by Eartha Kitt with Henri Rene & His Orchestra
47 **We Need a Little Christmas** by Johnny Mathis
58 **Santa Claus is Coming to Town** by Dolly Parton
71 **A Holly Jolly Christmas** by Alan Jackson
13 **Rockin' Around the Christmas Tree** by Brenda Lee
17 **Rudolph the Red Nosed Reindeer** by Burl Ives
42 **Last Christmas** by Wham!

HOME FOR THE HOLIDAYS
62 **Merry Christmas Everyone** by Shakin' Stevens
1 **Have Yourself a Merry Little Christmas**
by Vince Vance and The Valiants
26 **I Want a Hippopotamus for Christmas** by Gayla Peevey
18 **Mary's Boy Child** by Kensington Theatre Ensemble
73 **Honky Tonk Christmas** by Alan Jackson
63 **Winter Wonderland** by Brad Paisley
31 **Silent Night** by Kenny Vehkavaara

WHITE CHRISTMAS
31 **White Christmas** by Elvis Presley
34 **Let It Snow** by Papi Gonzales
25 **Winter Wonderland** by Engelbert Humperdinck
57 **Mele Kalikimaka** by Jimmy Buffet
2 **Christmas Cookies** by George Strait
66 **Jingle Bell Rock** by Bobby Helms
58 **You Make It Feel like Christmas**
by Gwen Stefani and Blake Shelton
43 **Let There Be Peace on Earth** by Bill & Gloria Gaither

BLUE CHRISTMAS
36 **Grandma Got Run Over by a Reindeer** by Elmo & Patsy
30 **Blue Christmas** by John Anderson
13 **All I Want for Christmas Is You**
by Vince Vance and The Valiants
58 **Santa Bring My Baby Back to Me** by Elvis Presley
46 **Last Christmas** by Glee Cast
17 **Please Daddy (Don't Get Drunk This Christmas)**
by Alan Jackson
53 **Pretty Paper** by Randy Travis

JAZZY CHRISTMAS
13 **Feliz Navidad** by Kenny Vehkavaara
61 **God Rest Ye Merry Gentlemen** by Kenny Vehkavaara
55 **Sleigh Ride** by Kenny Vehkavaara
54 **Jingle Bell Rock** by Jack Jezzro and Sam Levine
48 **Jingle Bells** by Kenny Vehkavaara
50 **Frosty the Snowman** by Kenny Vehkavaara
31 **The Christmas Song** by Kenny Vehkavaara
10 **White Christmas** by Kenny Vehkavaara
34 **Rockin' Around the Christmas Tree**
by Jack Jezzro and Sam Levine

THE DANCES BY THEIR STEPS

Basic: 7, 8, 9, 20, 24, 38, 47, 52, 55, 65, 67, 73

Behind-side-cross: 40, 44

Brush: 6, 14, 17, 28

Charleston: 2, 15, 24, 40

Coaster: 23, 32, 57, 58, 61

Conga Walk: 4, 18, 21, 34

Diagonal steps: 3, 6, 17, 20, 28, 33, 35, 60, 66, 70, 72, 75

Elvis knees: 69

Flick: 20

Heel Bounce: 54, 71

Hip bump: 14

Hitch/kick: 3, 4, 17, 18, 20, 21, 28, 34, 38, 39, 47, 49, 50, 52, 54, 56, 60, 70, 73

Jazz box: 6, 8, 11, 12, 16, 19, 20, 21, 22, 25, 27, 30, 33, 36, 39, 42, 51, 65, 66, 74

K-step: 18, 46, 62, 70, 71

Kick-ball-change: 1, 26, 52

Lindy: 8, 9, 21, 26, 30, 33, 37, 38, 39, 46, 47, 48, 52, 55, 56, 57, 59, 65, 66, 67, 74

Mambo: 13, 19, 22, 27, 32, 41, 50, 69

Merengue: 26, 34

Montana kick: 37, 70

Moon walk: 42, 48

Monterey turn: 21, 40, 59, 69

Pivot/paddle: 1, 3, 4, 5, 7, 9, 13, 15, 23, 25, 27, 31, 32, 37, 38, 42, 44, 45, 46, 51, 55, 57, 58, 60, 61, 62, 67, 70

Push step: 33

Rhumba: 5, 7, 10, 16, 22, 23, 27, 32, 34, 45, 50, 65, 69, 72

Rock-recover: 4, 5, 10, 11, 16, 19, 31, 34, 36, 45, 47, 50, 61, 62, 63, 66, 74

Rocking chair: 4, 5, 7, 13, 16, 24, 26, 30, 33, 37, 39, 42, 44, 47, 49, 52, 54, 55, 56, 67, 75

Sailor: 15, 61

Scuff: 37, 49, 52, 71

Shimmy: 73

Shuffle box: 1, 11, 12, 14, 30, 31, 55, 69

Scissors: 6, 17, 23, 35

Sway: 1, 25, 38, 60

Toe fan: 52, 73

Toe strut: 56

Triple step: 2, 10, 11, 12, 19, 23, 25, 26, 30, 31, 36, 39, 42, 44, 45, 46, 48, 49, 51, 58, 59, 60, 61, 62, 65, 74

V-step: 14, 20, 46, 54, 57, 61, 71

Vine: 2, 3, 4, 5, 6, 14, 16, 17, 18, 25, 28, 34, 36, 37, 47, 48, 51, 54, 66, 71, 75

Waltz steps (hesitation, twinkle, waltz, waltz box): 29, 41, 43, 53, 68

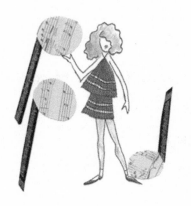

SONG INDEX

ARTIST INDEX

ABBA * I Do, I Do, I Do, I Do * Take a Chance on Me

The **Ad Libs** * Boy from NYC

Al **Alberts** and The Four Aces * Heart and Soul

Lily **Allen** * Dream a Little Dream (with Robbie Williams)

Herb **Alpert** & The Tijuana Brass * Bittersweet Samba *
Limbo Rock * This Guy's in Love with You

America * A Horse with No Name

American Patriots * Deep in the Heart of Texas

John **Anderson** * Blue Christmas * I'm Just an Old Chunk of Coal
* Swingin'

Lynn **Anderson** * Rose Garden

Chris **Andrews** * Pretty Belinda

The **Angels** * My Boyfriend's Back

Paul **Anka** * Diana * Pennies from Heaven (with Michael Buble)

The **Archies** * Sugar, Sugar

Louis **Armstrong** * A Kiss to Build a Dream on * In the Shade of
the Old Apple Tree (with The Mills Brothers) * Mame

Asleep at the Wheel * Get Your Kicks on Route 66

Fred **Astaire** * Cheek to Cheek

Chet **Atkins** * Alley Cat

Atlanta Rhythm Section * So into You

Gene **Autry** * Home on the Range

Frankie **Avalon** * Beauty School Dropout

David **Ball** * Swing Baby

The **Band Perry** * Gentle on My Mind

Bobby **Bare** * Detroit City * 500 Miles Away from Home

Len **Barry** * 1-2-3

Bart & Baker * Istanbul (Not Constantinople)

The **Beach Boys** * Dance, Dance, Dance * Don't Worry Baby *
Kokomo * Wouldn't It Be Nice

The **Bee Gees** * Stayin' Alive * To Love Somebody

Lou **Bega** * Mambo No. 5

Harry **Bellafonte** * Jamaica Farewell

The **Bellamy Brothers** * Almost Jamaica * Let Your Love Flow

Tony **Bennett** * On the Sunny Side of the Street
(with Willie Nelson)

Berlin * Take My Breath Away

Chuck **Berry** * School Day

Big Tom * The Same Way You Came In

Elvin **Bishop** * Fooled Around and Fell in Love

Stephen **Bishop** * On and On

Tia **Blake** * Plastic Jesus

Marcie **Blane** * Bobby's Girl

Bobby **Bloom** * Montego Bay

Boney M. * Mary's Boy Child

Booker T. & The M. G.'s * Green Onions

Pat **Boone** * Love Letters in the Sand

Bouke * A Love Worth Waiting for * Spanish Eyes

The **Box Tops** * The Letter

Ann **Breen** * It's a Sin to Tell a Lie

Brewer & Shipley * One Toke over the Line

Lane **Brody** * The Yellow Rose (with Johnny Lee)

Brooks & Dunn * My Maria * Neon Moon

Bobby **Brown** * Every Little Step * My Prerogative

Michael **Bublé** * All I Do Is Dream of You * All of Me * Pennies from Heaven (with Paul Anka)

Jimmy **Buffett** * Come Monday * Grapefruit – Juicy Fruit * Margaritaville * Meme Kalikimaka * Show Me the Way to Go Home * Volcano

Cindy **Bullens** * Freddy My Love

Floyd **Burton** * Rambling Rose

Glenn **Campbell** * Rhinestone Cowboy * Southern Nights

Freddy **Cannon** * Palisades Park

Captain & Tennille * Do That to Me One More Time

Eric **Carmen** * Hungry Eyes

Kim **Carnes** * Bette Davis Eyes

The **Carpenters** * There's a Kind of Hush * Top of the World

The **Cascades** * Rhythm of the Rain

Johnny **Cash** * Swing Low Sweet Chariot * Understand Your Man

Rosanne **Cash** * If You Change Your Mind * Seven Year Ache

Frank **Chacksfield** * Inishannon Serenade

The **Champs** * Tequila

Gene **Chandler** * Duke of Earl

Chayanne * Mariana Mambo

Cher * Welcome to Burlesque

Mark **Chesnutt** * Woman

The **Chiffons** * He's so Fine * One Fine Day

The **Chordettes** * Lollipop * Mr. Sandman

Eric **Church** * Drink in My Hand

Classics IV * Spooky

Richard **Clayderman** * Begin the Beguine

Patsy **Cline** * I Fall To Pieces * You Made Me Love You

Rosemary **Clooney** * People Will Say We're in Love
(with Bing Crosby)

The **Coasters** * Poison Ivy

Coldplay * Viva La Vida

Nat King **Cole** * L-O-V-E * Walkin' My Baby Back Home

Brian **Coll** * Believe Me If All Those Endearing Young Charms

Perry **Como** * Catch a Falling Star * Papa Loves Mambo

Confederate Railroad * Trashy Women

John **Conlee*** Rose Colored Glasses

Arthur **Conley** * Sweet Soul Music

The **Contours** * Do You Love Me

Sam **Cooke** * Another Saturday Night * Bring It On Home To Me *
The Riddle Song * This Little Light of Mine *
Twistin' the Night Away

Cream * Sunshine of Your Love

Creedence Clearwater Revival * Bad Moon Rising * Cotton
Fields * Have You Ever Seen the Rain * Proud Mary

The **Crests** * Sixteen Candles

The **Crew Cuts** * Sh Boom (Life Could Be a Dream)

Jim **Croce** * Bad Bad Leroy Brown

Bing **Crosby** * Everybody Loves My Baby * People Will Say We're
in Love (with Rosemary Clooney) * Yes Sir! That's My Baby

Pablo **Cruise** * I Go to Rio

Culture Club * Karma Chameleon

Billy **Currington** * Good Directions

Billy Ray **Cyrus** * Achy Breaky Heart

Charlie **Daniels** * This Little Light of Mine (with Brenda Lee)

Bobby **Darin** * Dream Lover * Mack the Knife

The **Dave Clark Five** * Because

Skeeter **Davis** * I Forgot More Than You'll Ever Know

Doris **Day** * Perhaps, Perhaps, Perhaps * Singin' in the Rain

DeBarge * Rhythm of the Night

The **Del-Vikings** * Come Go with Me

The **Desert Rose Band** * One Step Forward

Jackie **DeShannon** * Put a Little Love in Your Heart

The **Diamonds** * Little Darlin'

Dion * Runaround Sue * The Wanderer

Dire Straits * Walk of Life

The **Dixie Cups** * Chapel of Love

DJ BoBo (Peter René Baumann) * Chihuahua *
Everybody (with INNA)

Fats **Domino** * Blueberry Hill

The **Doobie Brothers** * Listen to the Music

Lee **Dorsey** * Working in the Coal Mine

Dr. Victor * If You Wanna Be Happy

The **Drifters** * Save the Last Dance for Me *
There Goes My Baby * Under the Boardwalk

Drifting Cowboys * Your Cheatin' Heart (with Hank Williams)

Drivin N Cryin * Straight to Hell

The **Dubliners** * Molly Malone

Dave **Dudley** * Six Days on the Road

The **Eagles** * One Of These Nights

Edison Lighthouse * Love Grows (Where My Rosemary Goes)

Elmo & Patsy * Grandma Got Run Over by a Reindeer

The **Emotions** * The Best of My Love

The **Everly Brothers** * All I Have to Do Is Dream * Bye, Bye Love * Cathy's Clown * Lucille * So Sad (To Watch Good Love Go Bad) * Wake Up Little Susie * Walk Right Back

Shelley **Fabares** * Johnny Angel

Faces * Ooh La La

Shep **Fields** & His Rippling Rhythm * A Little Bit Independent (with Gene Merlino and Diana Lee)

Firefall * You Are the Woman

Ella **Fitzgerald** * Goody, Goody

The **Fleetwoods** * Come Softly to Me

Eddie **Floyd** * Blood is Thicker than Water

Red **Foley** * Too Old to Cut the Mustard (with Ernest Tubb)

Radney **Foster** * Just Call Me Lonesome

The **Foundations** * Build Me Up Buttercup

Four Tops * Ain't No Woman (Like the One I've Got) * Baby I Need Your Loving * I Can't Help Myself (Sugar Pie, Honey Bunch) * Standing in the Shadows of Love * Walk Away Renee

Peter **Frampton** * Show Me the Way

Connie **Francis** * Everybody's Somebody's Fool * Who's Sorry Now

Lefty **Frizzell** * If You've Got The Money

Bill & Gloria **Gaither** * Let There Be Peace on Earth

Gale **Garnett** * We'll Sing in the Sunshine

Marvin **Gaye** * How Sweet It Is (To Be Loved By You)

Crystal **Gayle** * Don't It Make My Brown Eyes Blue

The **Geezinslaws** * Put Another Log on the Fire

General Johnson & The Chairmen of the Board * 39-21-46 * Give Me Just a Little More Time

Georgia **Gibbs** * Tweedle Dee

Don **Gibson** * Oh Lonesome Me * Sea of Heartbreak

Mickey **Gilley** * Room Full of Roses * True Love Ways

Jimmy **Gilmer** & The Fireballs * Sugar Shack

Girls From Mars * Bei Mir Bist Du Schon

Glee Cast * Last Christmas

Gliese * I'm Too Sexy for My Shirt

Gold Star Ballroom Orchestra * Unchained Melody

Papi **Gonzalez** * Let It Snow

Leslie **Gore** * It's My Party

Eydie **Gorme** * Amor (with Los Panchos) * Blame It on the Bossa Nova * Pretty Blue Eyes (with Steve Lawrence) * The Girl from Ipanema (with Steve Lawrence)

The **Grass Roots** * Sooner or Later

Al **Green** * Let's Stay Together

Norman **Greenbaum** * Spirit in the Sky

Lee **Greenwood** * Dixie Road

Daryl **Hall** & John Oates * Maneater

George **Hamilton** IV * Abilene * You Are My Sunshine

Albert **Hammond** * It Never Rains in Southern California

Ronan **Hardiman** * Dance Above the Rainbow

Emmylou **Harris** * C'est La Vie

Wilbert **Harrison** * Kansas City

Nancy **Hays** * Come Dance with Me

Bobby **Helms** * Jingle Bell Rock

Clarence "Frogman" **Henry** * (I Don't Know Why) But I Do

The **Highway Men** * Michael Row the Boat Ashore

Eddie **Hill** * Salty Dog Rag

Al **Hirt** * Java

The **Hollies** * He Ain't Heavy He's My Brother

Buddy **Holly** * Everyday * That'll Be the Day

Hollywood Argyles * Alley Oop

Rupert **Holmes** * Escape (the Pina Colada Song)

Dr. **Hook** * When You're in Love with a Beautiful Woman

Hot Chocolate * You Sexy Thing

Engelbert **Humperdinck** * After the Lovin' * Les Bicyclettes de Belsize * The Last Waltz * Winter Wonderland

Brian **Hyland** * Gypsy Woman

The **Impressions** * It's All Right

INNA (Elena Alexandra Apostoleanu) * Everybody (with DJ BoBo)

The **Isley Brothers** * This Old Heart of Mine (Is Weak for You)

Burl **Ives** * Rudolph the Red Nosed Reindeer

Alan **Jackson** * A Holly Jolly Christmas * In the Garden * Honky Tonk Christmas * How Great Thou Art * I Only Want You for Christmas * If You Don't Wanna See Santa Claus Cry * Meat and Potato Man * Please Daddy (Don't Get Drunk This Christmas)

Michael **Jackson** * Billie Jean * Butterflies * Rock with You * The Way You Make Me Feel

The **Jackson 5** * I Saw Mommy Kissing Santa Claus * Little Bitty Pretty One

The **Jacksons** * Blame It on the Boogie

Tony **Jackson** * It's Only Make Believe

Waylon **Jennings** * Good Hearted Woman

Jack **Jezzro** * Jingle Bell Rock (with Sam Levine) * Rockin' Around the Christmas Tree

Charles Johnson * It's Gonna Rain

George **Jones** * I Was Country When Country Wasn't Cool (with Barbara Mandrell)

Jimmy **Jones** * Handy Man

Tom **Jones** * Green Green Grass of Home

The **Judds** * Grandpa (Tell Me 'Bout The Good Old Days) * Rockin' with the Rhythm of the Rain

Ernie **K-Doe** * Mother-In-Law

Israel Ka'ano'i **Kamakawiwo'ole** * Over the Rainbow

Theo **Katzman** and Vulfpeck * Lonely Town

KC & The Sunshine Band * Get Down Tonight

The **Kendalls** * Heaven's Just a Sin Away

Chris **Kenner** * I Like It Like That

Kensington Theatre Ensemble * Mary's Boy Child

Andy **Kim** * Rock Me Gently

Ben E. **King** * Spanish Harlem * Stand by Me

Carole **King** * It's Too Late

The Nicol **Kings** * Exes and Ohs

The **Kingsmen** * Louie Louie

Eartha **Kitt** * Santa Baby (with Henri Rene & His Orchestra)

Gladys **Knight** & The Pips * Midnight Train to Georgia

Lady Antebellum * Silver Bells

Cyndi **Lauper** * Girls Just Want to Have Fun

Steve **Lawrence** * Pretty Blue Eyes (with Eydie Gorme) *
The Girl from Ipanema (with Eydie Gorme)

Brenda **Lee** * Rockin' Around the Christmas Tree * Sweet Nothin's
* This Little Light of Mine (with Charlie Daniels)

Curtis **Lee** * Pretty Little Angel Eyes

Diana **Lee** * A Little Bit Independent
(with Gene Merlino and Shep Fields & His Rippling Rhythm)

Johnny **Lee** * Red Sails in the Sunset *
The Yellow Rose (with Lane Brody)

Peggy **Lee** * Big Spender * It's a Good Day

Scooter **Lee** * Fly Me to the Moon * Here Lately *
Roll Back the Rug

Sam **Levine** * Jingle Bell Rock (with Jack Jezzro)

Little Milton * The Blues Is Alright

Little River Band * Reminiscing

LOCASH * Love Drunk

Hank **Locklin** * Please Help Me, I'm Falling

Loggins & Messina * Your Mama Don't Dance

Guy **Lombardo** * Enjoy Yourself (It's Later Then You Think) *
Five Foot Two Eyes of Blue

Julie **London** * Me and My Shadow

Looking Glass * Brandy

Los Panchos * Amor (with Eydie Gorme)

Lyle **Lovett** * You've Got a Friend in Me (with Randy Newman)

Patty **Loveless** * If My Heart Had Windows

Frankie **Lymon** & The Teenagers * Why Do Fools Fall in Love

Loretta **Lynn** * Coal Miner's Daughter

Major Dundee Band * Sweet Little Liza (with Dick Van Altena)

The **Mamas & The Papas** * California Dreamin' * Dream a Little
Dream of Me

Melissa **Manchester** * Midnight Blue

Henry **Mancini** * Pink Panther Theme

Barbara **Mandrell** * I Was Country When Country Wasn't Cool (with George Jones)

Barry **Manilow** * Copacabana (At the Copa) * Fugue for Tinhorns

Barry **Mann** * Who Put the Bomp

Bob **Marley** & The Wailers * Buffalo Soldier * Is This Love * One Love/People Get Ready * Three Little Birds

Bruno **Mars** * Uptown Funk (with Mark Ronson)

Little Peggy **Marsh** * I Will Follow Him

Dean **Martin** * Ain't That a Kick in the Head * C'est Magnifique * I Wonder Who's Kissing Her Now * On the Street Where You Live * You're Nobody 'til Somebody Loves You

Al **Martino** * Fascination

The **Marvelettes** * Please Mr. Postman

Johnny **Mathis** * We Need a Little Christmas

Kathy **Mattea** * Eighteen Wheels and A Dozen Roses

Frankie **McBride** * Could I Have This Dance

Helen **McCaffrey** * I'll Get Over You

Sir Paul **McCartney** * I'm Gonna Sit Right Down and Write Myself a Letter

Mel **McDaniel** * Louisiana Saturday Night

Gene **McDaniels** * A Hundred Pounds of Clay

Reba **McEntire** * Amazing Grace

Bobby **McFarrin** * Don't Worry, Be Happy

Tim **McGraw** * Just to See You Smile

The **McGuire Sisters** * Bye Bye Blackbird * 'S Wonderful *
Something's Gotta Give * Tip Toe Through the Tulips

Johnny **Mercer** * Baby It's Cold Outside (with Margaret Whiting) *
Summer Wind

Gene **Merlino** * A Little Bit Independent
(with Diana Lee and Shep Fields & His Rippling Rhythm)

Michael Learns To Rock * Blue Night

Heather **Miles** * Who Did You Call Darlin'

Bette **Midler** * Mambo Italiano

Glenn **Miller** * In the Mood

Mitch **Miller** * I'm Looking over a Four Leaf Clover

Roger **Miller** * Billy Bayou * Engine, Engine #9 * King of the Road

The **Mills Brothers** * Between Winston-Salem and Nashville
Tennessee * Cab Driver * Glow Worm * I've Got My Love to Keep
Me Warm * In the Shade of the Old Apple Tree (with Louis
Armstrong) * Nevertheless (I'm in Love with You) * Release Me *
Till Then * Tiny Bubbles * (Up A) Lazy River

Ronnie **Milsap** * (There's) No Getting' Over Me

Miss Rose and Her Rhythm Percolators *
Button Up Your Overcoat

Lorrie **Morgan** * Except for Monday

Jason **Mraz** * I'm Yours

Moon **Mullican** * I'll Sail My Ship Alone

Mungo Jerry * In the Summertime

Michael Martin **Murphey** * Land of Enchantment

Anne **Murray** * All I Have to Do Is Dream * Are You Lonesome Tonight * Don't Get Around Much Anymore * I Wonder Who's Kissing Him Now * Make Love to Me * There Goes My Everything

Johnny **Nash** * I Can See Clearly Now

Ricky **Nelson** * Garden Party * Poor Little Fool

Willie **Nelson** * A Fool Such as I (with Hank Snow) * On the Road Again * On the Sunny Side of the Street (with Tony Bennett)

The **New Summer Fun Project** * Girl Watcher

The **Newbeats** * Bread & Butter

Randy **Newman**
You've Got a Friend in Me (with Lyle Lovett)

Wayne **Newton**
Danke Schoen

Olivia **Newton-John** * Hopelessly Devoted to You * Summer Nights (with John Travolta) * You're the One That I Want (with John Travolta)

Harry **Nilsson** * Coconut * Everybody's Talkin' *
I Wonder Who's Kissing Her Now

Nitty Gritty Dirt Band * An American Dream * Fishin' in the Dark * Jambalaya (On The Bayou)

Chris **Norman** * Gypsy Queen

The **O Jays** * Love Train

Anita **O'Day** * It's Delovely

Kelli **O'Hara** * Honey Bun

The **Oak Ridge Boys** * Elvira * Y'all Come Back Saloon

Ocean * Put Your Hand in the Hand

Danny **Ocean** * Veneno

Luca **Olivieri** * She's Not You

The **Olympics** * (Baby) Hully Gully

Omar and The Howlers * Hit the Road, Jack

Roy **Orbison** * Only the Lonely * Uptown * You Got It

Tony **Orlando** and Dawn * Candida *
Who's in the Strawberry Patch with Sally

Orleans * Dance with Me * Still the One

K. T. **Oslin** * Do Ya'

Buck **Owens** * Act Naturally * I've Got a Tiger by the Tail *
Streets of Bakersfield

Patti **Page** * Tennessee Waltz * Try to Remember

Brad **Paisley** * Winter Wonderland

Dolly **Parton** * Islands in the Stream (with Kenny Rogers) *
Santa Claus is Coming to Town

The **Partridge Family** * I Think I Love You

Gayla **Peevey** * I Want a Hippopotamus for Christmas

Belle **Perez** * Amame

Wilson **Pickett** * Mustang Sally

Pink Martini * Bitty Boppy Betty

The **Platters** * Only You (And You Alone) * The Great Pretender *
Twilight Time

Player * Baby Come Back

The **Pointer Sisters** * I'm so Excited

The **Police** * Every Breath You Take

The **Poni-Tails** * Born Too Late

Ricchi E **Poveri** * Mamma Maria

Elvis **Presley** * Burning Love * It's Now or Never * Santa Bring My
Baby Back to Me * Santa Claus is Back in Town * Steamroller
Blues * White Christmas

Lloyd **Price** * I'm Gonna Get Married * Lady Luck *
No If's – No And's * Personality * Stagger Lee

Eddie **Rabbitt** * I Love a Rainy Night

Eddy **Raven** * I Got Mexico

The **Rays** * Silhouettes

Otis Redding * (Sittin' on) the Dock of the Bay

Jim **Reeves** * Across the Bridge * He'll Have to Go *
Take My Hand, Precious Lord

Martha **Reeves** & The Vandellas * Dancing in the Street *
Jimmy Mack

REO Speedwagon * Silent Night

Lionel **Richie** * Penny Lover

Jeannie C. **Riley** * Harper Valley P.T.A.

Johnny **Rivers** * Poor Side of Town

Marty **Robbins** * A White Sport Coat (and A Pink Carnation)

Smokey **Robinson** & The Miracles * I Second That Emotion *
Shop Around * The Tracks of My Tears

Kenny **Rogers** * Island in the Stream (with Dolly Parton)

Roy **Rogers** * Don't Fence Me In * Happy Trails (with Dale Evans) * The Yellow Rose of Texas

The **Rolling Stones** * Beast of Burden * Paint It, Black

The **Ronettes** * Be My Baby

Mark **Ronson** * Uptown Funk (with Bruno Mars)

Linda **Ronstadt** * Blue Bayou * I Can't Help It If I'm Still in Love with You * Just One Look

Darius **Rucker** * Wagon Wheel

Jimmy **Ruffin** * What Becomes of the Brokenhearted

Bobby **Rydell** * Forget Him

SSGT Barry **Sadler** * The Ballad of the Green Berets

Kyu **Sakamoto** * Sukiyaki

Sam & Dave * Soul Man

Sam The Sham & The Pharaohs * Lil Red Riding Hood

Santana * Adouma * Do You Remember Me * Game of Love (with Tina Turner) * In Search of Mona Lisa

Boz **Scaggs** * I'm a Fool to Care

The **Searchers** * Needles and Pins

Neil **Sedaka** * Breaking Up is Hard to Do * Oh Carol * Calendar Girl

The **Seekers** * I'll Never Find Another You

Del **Shannon** (Charles Weedon Westover) * Poor Side of Town * Runaway

Blake **Shelton** * Ready to Roll * Some Beach *
You Make It Feel like Christmas (with Gwen Stefani)

The **Shirelles** * Soldier Boy * Will You Love Me Tomorrow

Shirley & Lee * Let the Good Times Roll

Carly **Simon** * Mockingbird (with James Taylor) * You're so Vain

Jessica **Simpson** * What Christmas Means to Me

Frank **Sinatra** * Ain't She Sweet * Anything Goes * I've Got You
Under My Skin * Love is Here to Stay * Somethin' Stupid (with
Nancy Sinatra) * The Way You Look Tonight * Theme from
New York, New York * You Make Me Feel so Young

Nancy **Sinatra** * Somethin' Stupid (with Frank Sinatra) *

The **Singing Nuns** * Dominique

Ricky **Skaggs** * Highway 40 Blues

Lynyrd **Skynyrd** * Sweet Home Alabama

Sammi **Smith** * Help Me Make It Through the Night

Hank **Snow** * A Fool Such as I (with Willie Nelson)

The **South Street Band** * You Make My Dreams Come True

The **Spinners** * I'll Be Around * Working My Way Back to You

Squirrel Nut Zippers * Hey Shango! * Pay Me Now (or Pay Me
Later) * Put a Lid on It

Terry **Stafford** * Suspicion

Stargazers * The Vatican Rag

Starland Vocal Band * Afternoon Delight

Kay **Starr** * The Rock and Roll Waltz

Ringo **Starr** * It Don't Come Easy * No No Song *
Only You (And You Alone)

Starship * Nothing's Gonna Stop Us Now

The **Statler Brothers** * Do You Remember These? *
Flowers on the Wall * Oh Baby Mine (I Get so Lonely)

Gwen **Stefani** * You Make It Feel like Christmas (with Blake
Shelton)

Dodie **Stevens** * Pink Shoe Laces

John **Stevens** * It Had to Be You * My Blue Heaven

Ray **Stevens** * Everything is Beautiful

Shakin **Stevens** * Merry Christmas Everyone

Rod **Stewart** * Maggie May

George **Strait** * All My Exes Live in Texas * Christmas Cookies *
I Just Want to Dance with You * Milk Cow Blues * One Night at a
Time * Right or Wrong * The Chair * You Look so Good in Love

Marty **Stuart** * Western Girls

The **Stylistics** * I'm Stone in Love with You

Donna **Summer** * Hot Stuff

The **Supremes** * Love is Here and Now You're Gone *
Stop! In the Name of Love * Where Did Our Love Go

Billy **Swan** * I Can Help

Sylvia * Nobody

James **Taylor** * Mockingbird (with Carly Simon) *
You've Got a Friend

The **Teenagers** * Why Do Fools Fall in Love

The **Temptations** * Ain't Too Proud to Beg * Just My Imagination (Running Away with Me) * My Girl * Some Enchanted Evening

Three Degrees * When Will I See You Again

Three Dog Night * Joy to the World * Shambala

Johnny **Tillotson** * Listen to the Rhythm of the Falling Rain * Poetry in Motion * Red Roses for a Blue Lady

The **Tokens** * The Lion Sleeps Tonight (Wimoweh)

The **Tractors** * Pick Me Up on Your Way Down

Train * Hey, Soul Sister * Play That Song

Randy **Travis** * Forever and Ever Amen * Meet Me Under the Mistletoe * On the Other Hand * Pretty Paper

John **Travolta** * Sandy * Summer Nights (with Olivia Newton-John) * You're the One That I Want (with Olivia Newton-John)

Travis **Tritt** * Here's a Quarter (Call Someone Who Cares)

Doris **Troy** * Just One Look

Ernest **Tubb** * Too Old to Cut the Mustard (with Red Foley) * Waltz Across Texas

Josh **Turner** * Why Don't We Just Dance

Tina **Turner** * Game of Love (with Santana) * What's Love Got to Do with It

The **Turtles** * Happy Together

Conway **Twitty** * Hello Darlin' * It's Only Make Believe

Bonnie **Tyler** * It's a Heartache

Frankie **Valli** * Grease * Let's Hang On * Rag Doll

Frankie **Valli** & The Four Seasons * Big Girls Don't Cry *
December, 1963 (Oh What A Night) * Sherry * Walk like a Man

Dick **Van Altena** * Sweet Little Liza (with Major Dundee Band)

Ricky **Van Shelton** * Don't We All Have The Right *
From a Jack to a King

Vince **Vance** & The Valiants * All I Want for Christmas is You *
Have Yourself a Merry Little Christmas

Bobby **Vee** * Take Good Care of My Baby

Kenny **Vehkavaara** * Feliz Navidad * Frosty the Snowman *
God Rest Ye Merry Gentlemen * Jingle Bells * Silent Night *
Silver Bells * Sleigh Ride * The Christmas Song *
White Christmas * Winter Wonderland

Bobby **Vinton** * Beer Barrel Polka * Pennsylvania Polka

Theo Katzman and **Vulfpeck** * Lonely Town

John **Waite** * Missing You

Clay **Walker** * Blue Christmas

Jr. **Walker** & The All Stars * Shotgun

Gene **Watson** * Fourteen Carat Mind *
Got No Reason Now For Goin' Home

Mary **Wells** * My Guy * You Beat Me to the Punch

Matthew **West** * Hello My Name Is

Wham! * Last Christmas

Margaret **Whiting** * Baby It's Cold Outside (with Johnny Mercer)

Keith **Whitley** * Don't Close Your Eyes

Don **Williams** * I Believe in You * It Must be Love * Tulsa Time

Hank **Williams** * Hey Good Lookin' * I'm so Lonesome I Could Cry * Lovesick Blues * Move It on Over * Take These Chains from My Heart * There's a Tear in My Beer (with Hank Williams, Jr.) * Your Cheatin' Heart (with Drifting Cowboys)

Hank **Williams**, Jr. * Ain't Misbehavin' * Family Tradition * There's a Tear in My Beer (with Hank Williams) * Whiskey Bent and Hell Bound

Maurice **Williams** & The Zodiacs * Stay

Robbie **Williams** * Dream a Little Dream (with Lily Allen)

Jackie **Wilson** * That's Why (I Love You So)

Stevie **Wonder** * A Place in the Sun * Signed, Sealed, Delivered (I'm Yours) * Uptight (Everything's Alright)

Tammy **Wynette** * Stand by Your Man

Faron **Young** * Hello Walls

Paul **Young** * Every Time You Go Away

Zac Brown Band * Island Song

The **Zombies** * She's Not There

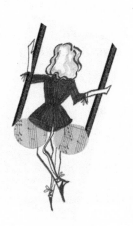

Made in the USA
Las Vegas, NV
22 January 2023

66064603R00114